THE COMPLETE GUIDE TO

Stretching

Christopher M. Norris

A & C Black • London

| Note |
| Whilst every effort has been made to ensure that the content of this book is as technically accurate and as sound as possible, neither the editors nor the publishers can accept responsibility for any injury or loss sustained as a result of the use of this material. |

Published in 1999 by
A & C Black (Publishers) Ltd
35 Bedford Row, London WC1R 4JH

Previously published in 1994
as *Flexibility: Principles & Practice*

ISBN 0 7136 4956 9

A CIP catalogue record for this book
is available from the British Library.

Acknowledgements
Cover photograph courtesy of Jump, Hamburg.
Line diagrams by Ron Dixon of Techtype
and Jean Ashley.

Typeset in 10½ on 12pt Palatino

Printed and bound in Great Britain
by Biddles Ltd, Guildford and Kings Lynn

Contents

Preface

When we think of fitness, there is a tendency to focus firstly on stamina because of the associated benefits to the heart and circulation, and secondly on muscle toning for its effects on general body appearance – the slim, toned, physique being very fashionable. But flexibility is of vital importance, for the health of the musculo-skeletal system in particular. This often neglected element of an all-round fitness programme can reduce the chance of injury in sport and can lessen the pain which can result from postural problems in daily life.

This book's predecessor, *Flexibility: Principles and Practice*, was well received because it combined science and practice to come up with safe and effective exercises. *The Complete Guide to Stretching* takes this approach still further by increasing the depth of the scientific background which precedes the prescription of exercise, by introducing new information on muscle imbalance, and by detailing the latest stretching research. In addition, the number of exercises has been more than tripled to provide a wider variation of movements to choose from, so making the individualisation of a training programme more effective.

The change from photographs to line drawings to illustrate the individual exercises has led to an improvement in clarity of body positions, and the inclusion of references from scientific journals will improve the educational value of the book, enabling students on both exercise-related and therapy-related courses to follow up material.

Throughout this book individuals are referred to as 'he'. This should, of course, be taken to mean 'he' or 'she' where appropriate.

Chris Norris

The Scientific Principles behind Stretching

Chapter 1

Biomechanical Factors in Stretching

The study of the effect of mechanical forces on biological materials is known as *biomechanics*. Biomechanical principles are important to all aspects of sports training, but especially to stretching. To be effective, and to prevent injury, stretching exercises must be applied on a foundation of good biomechanical principles.

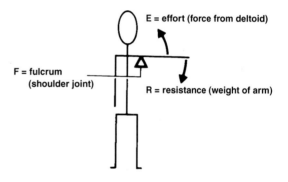

Figure 1.1 Leverage as the arm is abducted

♦ Leverage ♦

The limbs and spine act as *levers* when we move. A lever is simply a rigid bar which moves around a fixed point called the *pivot* or *fulcrum*. Two forces act on the lever, *effort* and *resistance*. The effort tries to move the lever, while the resistance tries to stop movement. In the body, the effort is supplied by muscle contraction, while the resistance is weight. The weight is a combination of the weight of the moving limb and the weight of any object lifted. Take as an example the arm lifting from the side of the body (*see* fig. 1.1). The fulcrum is the shoulder joint, the effort is supplied by the deltoid muscle, which contracts and abducts the arm, and the resistance is the weight of the arm.

How do you calculate the amount of leverage?

The amount of leverage produced in any exercise can be calculated by multiplying the weight of the resistance by the horizontal distance between the point where the resistance or effort acts and the fulcrum. Figure 1.2 illustrates a simple example of a lever. A resistance of 6 kg is placed 3 m away from the fulcrum. Multiplying these together gives a leverage force of 18 units. To balance this out, the effort has to be of the same magnitude. So, the 9 kg weight has to be placed only 2 m from the fulcrum for the lever to balance.

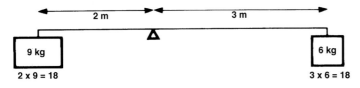

Figure 1.2 *Calculating leverage*

Leverage in stretching exercises

It is important to note that in the example given in figure 1.2 the horizontal distance between the fulcrum and effort or resistance is used, rather than simply the distance along the lever. This means that leverage will be increased as a body-part is moved into a horizontal position, and will reduce as the body-part moves away from the horizontal position (*see* fig. 1.3). This fact must always be borne in mind when choosing starting positions for stretching exercises, especially with regard to

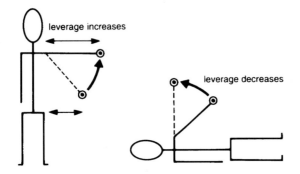

Figure 1.3 *Leverage in weight training*

injury to the spine. Take as an example a simple toe-touching movement. Performed from long sitting, the leverage on the spine is minimal (*see* fig. 1.4(a)); however, the same body movement performed from standing (*see* fig. 1.4(b)) places a considerable stress on the spine through leverage forces acting on the lumbar region.

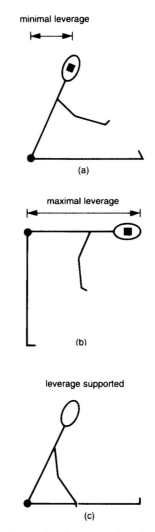

Figure 1.4 *Reducing leverage by altering the starting position*

This example illustrates an important safety factor with regard to leverage: exercises which involve moving the spine into a horizontal position will place great amounts of leverage on the spine and should be used with caution. Often, simply altering the starting position will move the spine away from the horizontal and reduce the stress on the lower back. When a horizontal position must be used, the spine should be supported. In the examples in figure 1.4, the athlete is stretching the hamstrings by bending forwards. This action places an excessive leverage stress on the spine. Simply by putting one hand down on the knee, the spine is supported and the stress reduced (*see* fig. 1.4(c)).

Considering the effect of *gravity* is also important. In figure 1.5 the athlete is performing the splits. The leverage on the leg is excessive, tending to force the knee downwards which opens the joint. This action can severely stress the medial ligament on the inside of the knee. Performing a similar action sitting down takes the weight away from the knee and, although the lever length is the same, the effect on the knee ligaments is considerably reduced, making the exercise far safer.

♦ Centre of gravity and ♦ stability

The *centre of gravity* of an object is its balance point, where all the weight of the object is focused. The centre of gravity of a symmetrical object, such as a brick, will be at its centre. However, in the case of asymmetrical objects, such as the human body, the centre of gravity will be nearer to the larger, and heavier, end.

Where is the body's centre of gravity?

Because the legs are heavier than the arms, when a person is standing their centre of gravity is not in the middle of the body at the naval, but lower down within the sacrum. As the body moves away from the standard upright position, the centre of gravity also moves. Lifting the arms overhead, for example, moves the centre of gravity upwards; while carrying something moves the centre of gravity towards the object being carried. In addition to the centre of gravity of the body as a whole, each limb also has a centre of gravity. For example, the weight of the arm will act through its own centre of gravity, which, rather

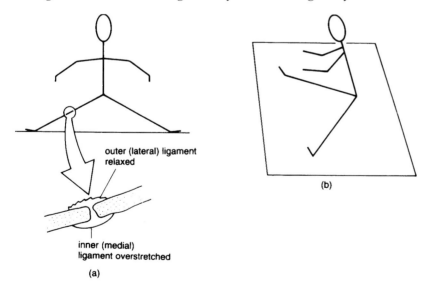

Figure 1.5 Leverage and the splits: (a) knees unsupported; (b) knees supported

outer (lateral) ligament relaxed

inner (medial) ligament overstretched

(a)

(b)

3

than being in the middle of the arm at the elbow, is actually closer to the shoulder because the upper arm is heavier than the forearm.

What affects stability?

Extending the centre of gravity downwards towards the floor gives us the object's *line of gravity*. Where the centre of gravity is the balance point of an object, the line of gravity can be imagined as a plumb-line hanging down from this point. For an object to remain in balance, its line of gravity must pass through its *base of support*. If the line of gravity moves outside the base of support, the object becomes unstable and will topple over. To compensate for this, the body position will change when something is carried. In figure 1.6(a) the centre of gravity of the body is within the sacrum. In figure 1.6(b), the suitcase carried in the right hand moves the centre of gravity of the body and case combined to the right. This would move the line of gravity outside the person's base of support, making him unstable. To compen-

sate for this the body position is changed, by leaning over to the left, to pull the line of gravity back within the base of support (*see* fig. 1.6(c)).

Stability is an important safety factor when performing stretching exercises. An unstable position can cause an athlete to wobble or fall, unintentionally increasing a stretch and pulling muscles or spraining joints. When discussing stability, there are two factors to consider: first, the position of the object's centre of gravity; and second, the size of the object's supporting base.

A lower centre of gravity and a wider base of support will make an object more stable. In addition, the degree of stability is proportional to the distance from the line of gravity to the outer limits of the base of support. Take as an example a motorbike (*see* fig. 1.7(a)). It has narrow wheels and thus a small base of support. In addition, the rider sits on the machine so his centre of gravity is high. If the rider were to lean over when going round a bend, he would become less stable (*see* fig. 1.7(b)). His base of support is the same, and his height above the ground is roughly the same, but his line of gravity has now moved

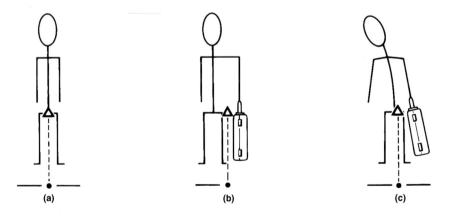

(a)   (b)   (c)

Figure 1.6 The centre of gravity of the body moves when an object is carried: (a) line of gravity through base of support = STABLE; (b) line of gravity moves outside base of support = UNSTABLE; (c) body shifts to bring line of gravity back within base = STABLE

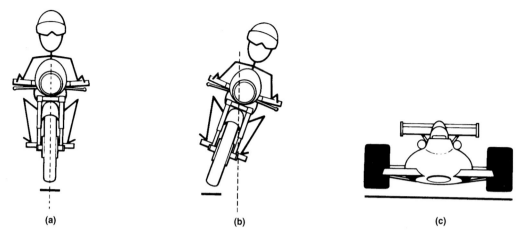

Figure 1.7 Stability, centre of gravity and base of support: (a) motorcycle upright – line of gravity midway through base; (b) motorcycle tipped – line of gravity at edge of base; (c) racing car – wide base of support

closer to the edge of his base of support. The motorcycle-rider's position is much less stable than that of a racing-car driver where the car has a wide base of support (*see* fig. 1.7(c)) and, because the driver sits low in the car rather than on top of it, the centre of gravity is lower.

How do you increase stability in an exercise?

The principles described above can be applied to the exercise situation. When performing standing exercises the centre of gravity is fairly high, so the feet should be apart to widen the base of support, which will make the position more stable. In addition, bending the knees will lower the centre of gravity and further increase stability. When moving, the base of support should be widened in the direction of the movement, i.e. when swinging the arms forwards and backwards a wide stance should be taken with one foot in front of the other, and when moving the arms from side to side the feet should be astride.

◆ Inertia, friction and ◆ momentum

Inertia

Inertia is an object's resistance to change in motion, and is proportional to its weight or 'mass'. Inertia is the force which makes a car hard to push, but a bicycle easy. The heavier an object is, the more inertia it will have. Once inertia has been overcome and the object has begun to move, less force is required to keep it in motion. This is why a heavy object may need a 'good push' to get it moving, and then as it starts to move it does so with a sudden jolt and seems to 'run away with itself'.

A joint possesses a certain inertia due to the stiffness (viscosity) of its synovial fluid, and the extensibility of the tissues (ligaments and muscles) which surround it. The first part of any movement sequence will often be the most difficult because it is overcoming joint inertia. Once the movement is 'going', keeping it going is often easier. The first action in any set of stretches can be seen as a warm-up, and each subsequent movement will gradually increase in range. In addition, a warm joint will offer less resistance to movement in general, and its inertia will be less. A warm-up before stretching, or any sport that involves range of motion exercise, is therefore important.

Friction

Friction, on the other hand, is the force which tries to stop one object from sliding over another. Frictional forces are the result of roughness on the surfaces of two opposing objects and can be reduced with the use of a lubricant like oil or water. On a rubberised floor the roughness of the floor and the sole of the shoe produces a large amount of friction and gives considerable grip. A shiny wooden floor produces less friction, and a patch of water will reduce friction still further and may cause a person to slip and fall.

Momentum

Momentum is the combination of how heavy an object is and how quickly it is moving (mass and velocity). A heavy object, such as a leg or the trunk, which is moving quickly will possess a lot of momentum and will be very difficult to stop. The high degree of momentum can take over the movement so that the athlete is no longer able to control it: this is when injuries can occur. To reduce the likelihood of injury through momentum, rapid actions should only be performed in mid-range. When going to full range, actions should be slow and controlled to avoid damage to the joint structures and to muscles. Momentum is a particularly important factor in ballistic stretching (*see* page 46).

◆ Tension, compression ◆ and shear

Tension, *compression* and *shear* are all examples of mechanical stresses which can act on the body, causing the body tissues to deform.

Tension is a pulling force. When the spine is flexed, the spinal ligaments are tightened and subjected to a tension stress that causes them to lengthen.

Compression stress is the opposite to tension stress. It is a pushing force, applied along the length of a tissue. When a person is standing upright the knee cartilages (menisci) take weight, and compression stress is applied to them, causing them to flatten.

Shear stress occurs when opposite forces are applied to a tissue, causing one part of the tissue to slide over the other. For example, if an athlete who is running stops suddenly by digging their foot into the ground, shearing stress is applied to the knee. Body-weight tries to keep the athlete moving forwards, but – because the foot is fixed on the ground – the ground force pushes in the opposite direction. The result of these two opposing forces is shear.

Mechanical stresses and injuries

Both compression and tension stresses act in line with the tissue fibres, in the direction in which the tissues are strongest. Shearing stresses, however, are imposed at an angle to the fibres, making this type of stress potentially the most dangerous in terms of injury. For example, a fall on to a straight leg will exert a compression stress on the joint structures. These forces will be largely absorbed, unless they are very severe. During the fall, tension stress will be imposed on the muscles if the joints bend, and the elastic capabilities of the muscles will take some of the stress away from the joint. Falling at an angle will again cause some compression and tension, but shearing will also take place between the body tissues and the foot and ground. This type of stress can cause injury, and a fracture may result.

♦ Tissue reaction to load ♦

The load–deformation curve

When a load is applied to a body tissue, the tissue will deform. The relationship between load (stress) and deformation (strain) can be represented graphically by the load–deformation curve (*see* fig. 1.8). Initially when the load is applied the tissue demonstrates elasticity. The deformation of the tissue at this point of the curve is directly proportional to the load which is applied (a relationship known as Hooke's law). As the load is released the tissue returns to its original shape – it literally 'bounces back'. To begin with, the amount of deformation is proportional to the load applied and there is said to be a *linear relationship* between load and deformation along this part of the curve called the *elastic range*.

If the load continues, the tissue is stretched beyond its elastic range and a point is reached at which deformation becomes permanent.

Past this point, known as the *elastic limit*, the tissue will not return to its original shape when the load is released, and a permanent change will occur. Instead of acting in an elastic fashion, the material is now said to be *viscous* or *plastic* in its reaction to load. The more load that is applied, the more deformed the material becomes. Instead of returning the load and bouncing back, the tissue is absorbing and dampening some of the load.

Eventually the yield point is reached, at the highest point of the curve. After this point the material continues to deform even though the load applied to it is not increasing; this means severe damage is occurring to the body tissue. This behaviour – continued deformation with constant load – is known as *creep*.

Properties of body tissues

Body tissues combine both viscous and elastic properties, so they are *viscoelastic*. One of the essential features of the deformation of viscoelastic materials is that it is time dependent. This means that when a load is applied rapidly (sudden stretch) the deformation will be elastic, and the tissue will spring back. If the load is applied for some time (stretch and hold) the deformation becomes viscous, and the tissue will slowly 'give'.

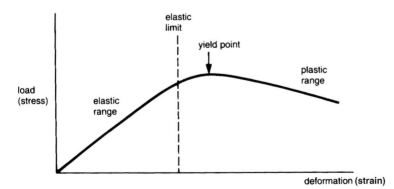

Figure 1.8 The load–deformation curve

◆ Composition and ◆ resolution of forces

Composition of forces

In figure 1.9(a) two men are pulling on ropes attached to a car bumper. Man A pulls at 45° to the car; man B also pulls at 45° but on the other side of the car. The net result is that the car rolls forwards. This process demonstrates the *composition of forces*. The forces supplied by the men pull at 90° to each other, combining to produce a third force – the *resultant* – which pulls the car forwards. A similar effect occurs in the body, where two muscles pull to create a third force. When the quadriceps muscles are pulling on the patella, the vastus medialis pulls inwards, and vastus lateralis pulls outwards. The result is a centrally directed pull of the kneecap. However, if one muscle is substantially stronger or tighter than the others, the direction of the patella will change and pain may result.

Resolution of forces

Where we have just one force, we can use the reverse process to obtain the two original forces which make up the resultant. Now we are using the process of *resolution of forces* to more accurately demonstrate the effect of the force on the body. For example, when someone who is running places their foot on the ground a force known as the *ground reaction force* is created. This acts obliquely to the ground (*see* fig. 1.9(b)). This single force may be resolved into its two components: one of which acts vertically to create compression or jarring stress on the foot; and one which acts horizontally causing shearing or friction on the foot.

Composition of forces in stretching exercises

The composition of forces can also be important when performing stretching exercises. Take as an example the quadriceps stretch

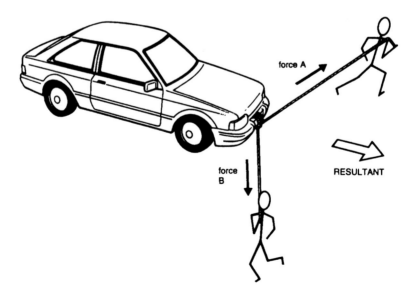

Figure 1.9(a) Forces A and B combine to produce the resultant, which pulls the car forwards

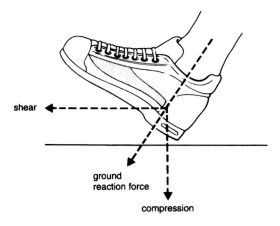

Figure 1.9(b) The ground reaction force has two components: shear and compression

(*see* page 89). As we bend the knee, the top of the patella is pulled upwards along the length of the femur and the patella tendon pulls downwards, in the opposite direction. The result is a composition of these two forces to create a third force compressing the patella on to the femur below. This action can be very painful in someone suffering from inflammation of the front of the knee (*see* fig. 1.10).

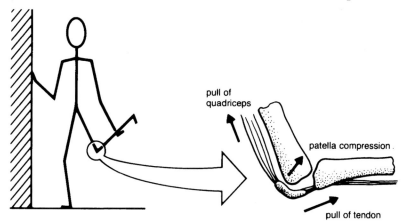

Figure 1.10 Patella compression can be very painful

◆ Describing body ◆ movement

Axes and planes

For descriptive purposes the human body may be divided into three planes. The *sagittal* plane passes through the body from front to back, dividing it into right and left halves. The *frontal* plane divides the body into anterior and posterior sections, and lies at right angles to the sagittal plane. The *transverse* plane divides the body into upper and lower portions, and rests at right angles to the other two planes.

Each of the three body planes has an associated axis which passes perpendicularly through it (*see* fig. 1.11). Movement occurs *in* a plane but *about* an axis. Abduction and adduction occur in the frontal plane about an anteroposterior (AP) axis; flexion and extension occur in a sagittal plane about a transverse axis; and rotations occur in a transverse plane about a vertical axis.

In reality, movements do not just occur in one plane, but in several. This is because a complex series of movements link together to give a motion that occurs in all three planes about an oblique axis.

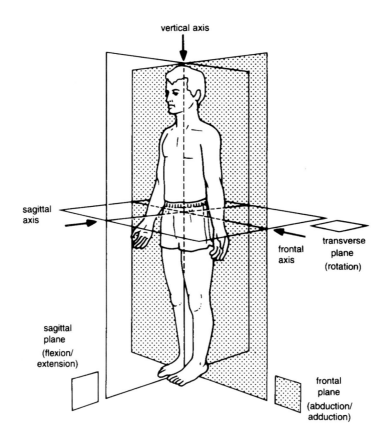

Figure 1.11 Axes and planes

Anatomical terminology

Standard terminology should be used when describing body movements to avoid confusion. For example, instead of 'bending' we use flexion, and instead of 'straightening' we use extension.

To describe the position of part of the body we again use standard terminology. So, instead of saying 'in front' we use the term anterior, and instead of 'above', the term superior is used.

Figure 1.12 shows the common terms used to describe movement and position of the body.

Range of motion

The range of motion (ROM) of a muscle refers to the length of the muscle at any point in a movement. *Outer range* is from a fully stretched position to the mid-point of the movement. *Inner range* is from this mid-point to a fully shortened position of the muscle. Mid-range is an area between these two extremes and is the region in which most everyday actions occur (*see* fig. 1.13).

It is important that the body tissues are regularly taken through their full range of motion to maintain their extensibility and elasticity. When this does not occur, the

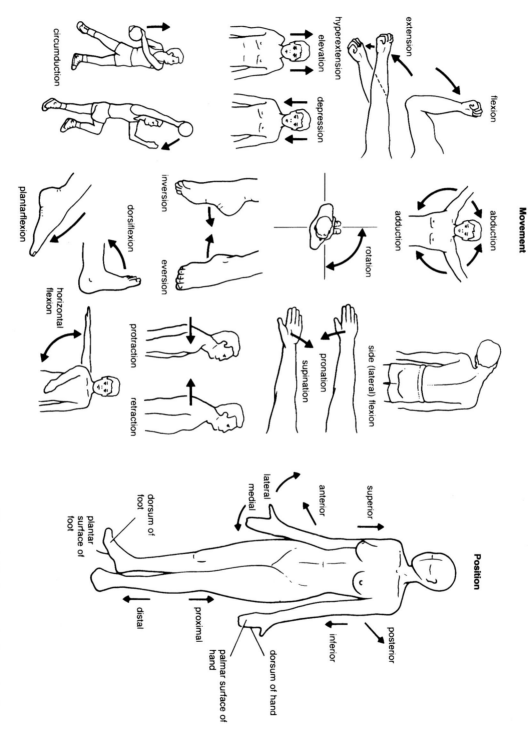

Figure 1.12 Anatomical terminology

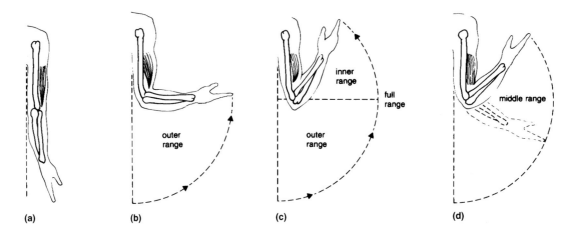

Figure 1.13 *Range of motion: (a) flexors of elbow fully extended; (b) flexors of elbow have moved through their outer range; (c) flexors of elbow have moved through their inner range; (d) flexors of elbow have moved within their middle range*

muscle can shorten permanently, completely altering the function of a joint. For example, in a sedentary individual it is common for the hip flexors to become shortened, because most everyday movements only work these muscles within their inner range. The shortened muscle may then pull on to the lumbar spine, giving back pain.

♦ Summary ♦

- A lever is a rigid bar which moves around a fixed point called the fulcrum.
- Leverage is calculated by multiplying the horizontal distance between the fulcrum and the line of action of a force acting on the lever.
- The centre of gravity of the body is near the sternum.
- As a body tissue is loaded, initially its reaction is elastic (it springs back) then plastic (it permanently deforms).
- Forces may be resolved into two components acting at 90° to each other.
- Motion may be outer, mid-, or inner range.

Chapter 2

Joint Structure and Function

♦ Bones ♦

The body has over 200 separate bones. Each is a rigid structure made from calcium, phosphorous and proteins. Bones may be divided into four major categories: long, short, flat and irregular.

- **Long** bones are the type found in the limbs such as the thigh (femur) and upper arm (humerus). Their primary use is to act as levers for the muscles to pull on when producing movement.
- **Short** bones are cube-shaped and seen in the carpels of the hand and tarsals of the forefoot.
- **Flat** bones, such as the scapulae and ribs, form broad areas for muscle attachment and serve to protect vital organs of the body.
- **Irregular** bones, such as the vertebrae, protect and support the body.

How do bones form?

Bone begins life as cartilage in the foetus. During the second month of pregnancy the cartilage bone begins to change into bone proper by a process known as *ossification* (*see* fig. 2.1). This begins in a primary centre in the middle of the bone and gradually spreads towards the bone-ends. This central portion of ossified bone is called the *diaphysis*, while the end of the bone which is still made of cartilage is the *epiphysis*. During adolescence a secondary ossification centre appears in the epiphysis. Ossification here spreads towards the shaft, leaving a thin cartilage growth plate (epiphyseal plate) sandwiched between the two regions of ossified bone.

How do bones grow?

The growth plate is responsible for change in the length of the bone. As a person reaches maturity, the epiphyseal plate will disappear and the shaft and extremity of the bone fuse into one solid unit. The epiphyseal plate is an area of potential weakness in the young bone, and if damaged can result in permanent deformity of the bone. This is especially true of the upper part of the femur in sport, and great care must be taken when giving stretching exercises to children so that excessive strain is not imposed on the hip.

What are bones made of?

As a long bone ossifies, its shaft becomes a cylinder with hard compact bone on the outside surrounding a central medullary cavity. The bone cavity contains bone marrow, responsible for making blood cells. The epiphysis is made from spongy cancellous bone with a thin compact bone covering. The other bone types do not contain a cavity but instead are made up of a honeycomb of

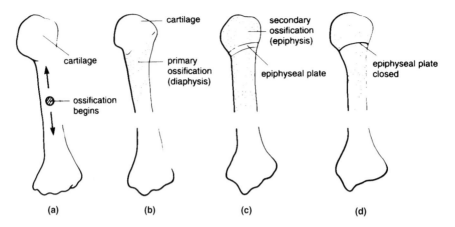

Figure 2.1 Ossification of centres in the bone: (a) embrionic; (b) infancy; (c) adolescence; (d) mature

cancellous bone with a thin compact bone covering. This makes them light although they may be bulky.

♦ Joint types ♦

In order for movement to occur in the body, the bones must articulate. The point at which this occurs is called a joint, and consists of two bones separated by various types of tissue. The shape of the bone-ends involved in a joint will dictate how much movement can occur, and which movement types are allowed. Joints may be broadly classified into three major groups, known as *fibrous* (immobile), *cartilaginous* (slightly mobile) and *synovial* (freely movable) (*see* table 2.1).

Fibrous joints

Fibrous joints allow little, if any, movement. Examples include the joints formed between the bones of the skull (a *suture* joint), those of the teeth (*gomphosis*), and *syndesmosis*, an example of which is found between the upper

end of the fibula and the upper outer aspect of the tibia.

The edges of the bones forming the suture joints of the skull are jagged and separated by fibrous tissue. This type of joint will not normally allow any perceptible movement, and may close up completely after the age of 30. The syndesmosis is also separated by fibrous tissue, but more than in the suture joint. The fibrous tissue in this joint forms a ligament which allows small amounts of twisting and stretching movements. The tooth joint, or gomphosis, consists of a peg which fits tightly into a socket and is held in place by a fibrous band.

Cartilaginous joints

In cartilaginous joints the bones are separated by a pad of cartilage tissue, and both primary and secondary types exist. The primary cartilaginous joint has articular cartilage separating the bones. They occur as the growth plates at the ends of bones in children. At the beginning of adult life the growth plate closes and the two pieces of bone (the diaphysis and epiphysis) become one bone. The secondary

Table 2.1 Joint types

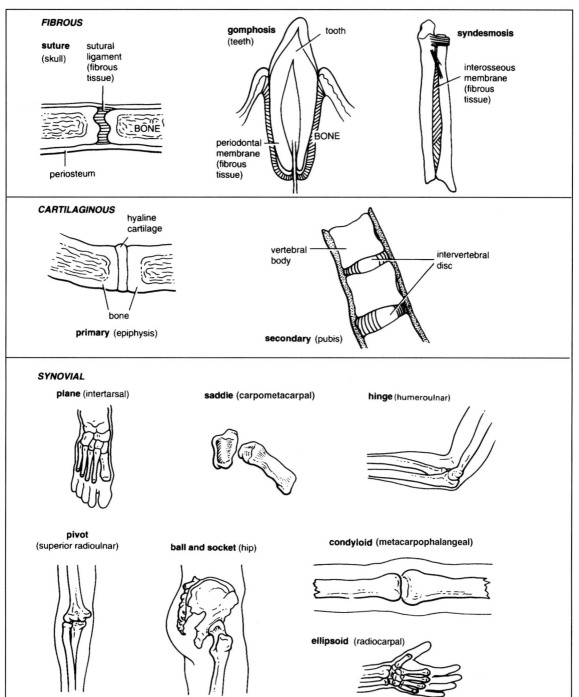

cartilaginous joints are found in the centre line of the body; examples include the spinal discs and the joint between the two pubic bones (known as the *symphysis pubis*). The bone-ends of the joint are separated from each other by a fibrocartilage pad, a structure which allows limited movement.

Synovial joints

The synovial joints are the ones we are most concerned with when using stretching exercises. They move freely and contain a variety of joint structures. A typical synovial joint consists of two bone-ends covered by articular cartilage.

The joint is surrounded by a fibrous joint capsule. Certain portions of the capsule are thickened to form supporting ligaments. The capsule is lined with a thin synovial membrane which secretes a lubricating liquid called *synovial fluid*. Structures inside the joint or within the capsule are known as *intra-capsular*. Structures associated with the joint but found outside the capsule are called *extra-capsular*. These include small balloon-like pads or *bursae* which stop structures rubbing over each other, and small 'fat pads' which fill the gaps between tissues.

Muscles control the joint, and those passing close to the bones may attach some fibres to the joint structures. For example, the popliteus muscle of the knee also attaches to the medial knee ligament and medial knee meniscus.

There are seven main types of synovial joints (*see* table 2.1).

- The **plane** joint has relatively flat surfaces and permits gliding or twisting of one bone against the other. The intertarsal joints of the foot are examples of plane joints.
- The **saddle** joint has one convex surface and one concave surface arranged at right angles to each other, as with a horse rider

sitting in a saddle. The major movements occur in two planes, with a slight amount of combined movement occurring in a third plane. An example is the carpometacarpal (CMC) joint of the thumb.

- The **hinge** joint allows movement in one axis only, and a strong joint is formed with tight ligaments. An example is the elbow joint (humeroulnar), formed between the humerus and ulna.
- The **pivot** joint allows a rotation movement about one axis only. One piece of bone rotates in a ring formed by the other bone and ligament tissue. An example is the joint formed between the radius and the ulna in the elbow (superior radioulnar).
- The **ball and socket** joint allows movement in all three planes, examples being the hip and shoulder joints. A ball-shaped surface of one bone articulates with a cup-shaped surface of the other.
- The **condyloid** joint is similar to the ball and socket, but allows movement in only two planes. The metacarpophalangeal (MCP) joints of the fingers are examples.
- The **ellipsoid** joint is again a modification of the ball and socket. The convex surface of one bone is oval in shape, while the concave surface of the opposing bone is elliptical. The radiocarpal joint in the wrist is an example here.

♦ Joint structures ♦

Individual differences in joint structures

Although each person has the same joint types, there is tremendous variation in the general structure and function of joints between two individuals.

The shapes of the bones will vary. This can be due to hereditary influences, physical training or injury. Some people are naturally more, or less, flexible because of the shapes of their bones.

Those who have exercised regularly since an early age will be considerably different from inactive individuals. For example, girls who have spent many years practising ballet as children will tend to be more flexible around the hips for the rest of their lives.

Injury and disease will also affect the range of motion which is possible at a joint. Older athletes who have varying amounts of arthritis will show reduced movement in specific patterns. For example, lateral rotation of the shoulder and hip tends to be very limited. Where an injury has occurred early in life the growth plate in a bone may have been affected. A severe fall from a bicycle or horse can often dislodge a bony growth plate and alter the formation of the final mature bone.

The structural differences at a joint must be appreciated when comparing ranges of movement between individuals. Even with the same amount of training, two people may never gain the same amount of movement at a joint.

Connective tissue and the formation of joint structures

The tissues of the body are of four basic types (*see* table 2.2). *Epithelial* tissue consists of densely packed cells which form coverings, and makes up skin and the outer coating of organs. *Connective* tissue is a fluid (described below) consisting of loosely arranged cells. *Muscular* tissue has the ability to contract, and *nervous* tissue to conduct electrical impulses.

Connective tissue consists of cells floating within a fluid known as an *extracellular matrix*. The composition of the cells and matrix determines the type and function of the particular connective tissue described. The cells have many functions including creating and main-

Table 2.2 Tissue types

Tissue	Function
Epithelial	Tightly packed cells which form coverings and make up skin and outer coating of organs.
Connective	Loose cells in fluid base which modify to form joint structures.
Muscular	Contracts muscles.
Nervous	Conducts electrical impulses.

taining the fluid matrix and ultimately breaking it down. Three types of fibres are found within the matrix. *Collagen* fibres are the most abundant and are so profuse that they may form one third of the total body-weight. The collagen fibres have a rope like appearance and are strong but non-elastic. The second type of fibre found is *elastin*. This resembles a coiled spring and has great elastic capacities. The elastin fibres crisscross each other to form a net, similar to the springs in a bed mattress. The third type of fibre is *reticular* fibre. Reticular fibres are really a type of collagen, and are very fine fibres which branch to form a meshwork.

The basic design of connective tissue is modified to form the various joint structures described below.

Types of joint structures

Articular cartilage
The ends of the bones forming a joint are covered by articular (hyaline) cartilage, a modified connective tissue. The cartilage matrix contains specialised cells known as *chondrocytes* which maintain its integrity. It also contains both collagen and elastin fibres in varying proportions together with proteoglycan, a protein which acts as a sponge to trap water, giving cartilage an exceptionally

high (70–80%) water content. Cartilage has no blood vessels or nerves, relying instead for its nutrition on the synovial fluid. Substances move into and out of the cartilage by diffusion from the synovial fluid, a process heavily reliant on regular movement to cause alterations in pressure within the fluid. As the cartilage is compressed intermittently with movement, for example walking or running, nutrients are pumped into and out of the cartilage. With continuous loading, such as occurs in prolonged standing, the cartilage is compressed further and further without allowing more fluid to be taken up. This continual compression without release can reduce the cartilage depth by as much as 40%.

The area of cartilage next to the bone (the sub-chondral region) is firmly attached to the bone and will resist shearing stresses. The main body of the cartilage contains fibres that will resist tension stresses, while the fluid within the cartilage gel resists compression stresses. The fibres are elastic, and the gel will gradually flow away from any compressing force. It is the combination of these two reactions that gives cartilage a viscoelastic property.

The joint capsule

The joint capsule is composed of two parts. The outer portion (stratum fibrosum) is tough and fibrous, and is thickened in certain areas to form ligaments. The inner portion of the capsule (stratum synoviale) is loose and contains many blood vessels. This region blends with the synovial membrane of the joint.

The capsule is attached to the bones around the edge of the joint, and at the line of attachments many small blood vessels are seen. The capsule has a rich supply of nerve fibres responsible for the 'joint sense' (proprioception) used in balance and reflex actions. The capsule is particularly important after injury. Following joint sprains, the joint will swell, and the accumulation of fluid will stretch the capsule causing tightness and pain. After injury the capsule can thicken and further limit the joint movement, requiring specialist physiotherapy techniques and regular stretching exercises to regain the lost movement.

Synovial membrane

The synovial membrane lines the joint capsule and consists of two distinct layers. The inner layer secretes the synovial fluid, while the outer layer is a loose, highly vascular structure consisting of collagen fibres and fat cells. This outer layer merges with the membrane covering the bones, the *periosteum*.

The blood vessels of the joint divide into three branches: one travelling to the epiphysis at the end of the bone; the second to the joint capsule; and the third to the synovial membrane itself. The blood vessels contained in the synovial membrane can exchange fluid and nutrient molecules with the synovial fluid. The synovial membrane has a series of folds in it and as the joint moves, it will unfold like a fan to allow movement (rather than simply stretching). The folds of the synovial membrane have extensive lubrication to virtually eliminate friction.

Ligaments

Many ligaments are simply parts of the joint capsule that have thickened to resist particular stresses on the joints. They are made of connective tissue fibres, and attach to the bones of the joint. The ligament fibres are arranged along the lines of stress imposed on the joint. As a joint moves the ligaments will stretch, initially pulling the fibres straight and then stretching them. Exercise will regularly lengthen the ligaments and strengthen them, but stretching exercises that overstress the ligaments should be avoided. The ligaments support the joint, and if overstretched can leave the joint too flexible, causing it to be insecure and open to injury. Following a ligament injury, it is particularly important to keep the joint moving gently, so that the newly healing ligament fibres will again align themselves correctly, rather than in a haphazard fashion.

Ligaments at the side of the joint (collateral ligaments) resist stresses which would tend to open the joint sideways. Other ligaments are positioned to protect the joint in its most vulnerable movements. For example, in the knee the cruciate ligaments prevent the thigh-bone (femur) from sliding forwards and backwards on the shinbone (tibia), and in the shoulder the glenohumeral ligament prevents the ball of the shoulder (head of humerus) from moving too far forwards in its socket (glenoid) and dislocating.

Consideration must be given to ligaments when stretching at all times. Stretches which are excessive or brutal in their application may actually damage the ligamentous support of a joint and cause severe injury.

Muscle–tendon unit

The muscles are attached to the bones via a tendon. This is an inelastic collagen structure that simply transmits the force created by the muscle to the bone in order to move it. The tendon is able to transmit the force to a small area, keeping the bulk of the muscle away from the joint. Some tendons, such as those of the finger muscles, are very long, allowing the muscles to be positioned in the forearm, well away from the finger joint where the muscle force is applied. Other tendons, such as that of the deltoid muscle of the shoulder, are right next to the muscle itself.

The thick, central part of the muscle is called the muscle belly, and it is this part which bulges as the muscle contracts. The muscle then tapers down towards the tendon and this area between the muscle and tendon is called the musculo-tendinous junction. The tendon then inserts into the bone via the teno-osseous junction.

Lubrication of joint cartilage

The articular cartilage has no blood supply. As we have seen, it relies largely for its nutrition on materials being passed from the synovial fluid. Movement will flush fresh fluid over the cartilage surface, and alterations in pressure will press nutrients into the cartilage. If the joint does not move properly, for example following injury, nutrient material may not be pressed into the cartilage, and that area may degenerate giving osteoarthritis.

The synovial fluid provides a lubricating mechanism which cuts down the amount of friction the joint is subjected to. As the two bony surfaces move over each other, the small synovial fluid molecules act as tiny ball-bearings preventing the opposing cartilage surfaces from rubbing away. Some of the fluid is absorbed into the cartilage almost like water in a sponge. As pressure is exerted on the joint, for example when standing or walking, the fluid is squeezed out of the cartilage forming a fluid film which separates the cartilage surfaces and again prevents them rubbing.

It is often said (usually by inactive individuals) that exercise causes arthritis. This is far from the case. Movement will actually keep the joint cartilage healthy and is essential for the general health of the joint. However, if an injury occurs and an athlete tries to 'train through the pain', the biomechanics of the joint will be altered and changes may occur in the joint cartilage, ultimately leading to the development of arthritis. In addition, a balance must be kept between the strength of muscles supporting a joint and the flexibility of the joint structures. If a person becomes too flexible the joint will not be secure. Similarly, if a person has too little flexibility their joints will be stiff. Either case will alter the normal biomechanics of a joint and could give problems later in life.

♦ Joint mechanics ♦

Physiological and accessory movements

Two major types of movement are possible at any joint. First, there are the normal actions which an athlete controls, such as flexion and extension. These are known as *physiological* movements. But there are also *accessory* movements, which cannot be produced directly but occur automatically as a joint moves, giving 'joint play'. For example, as the knee bends and straightens, the femur and tibia will also glide and roll on each other. The bending and straightening (flexion and extension) are the physiological movements, while the gliding and rolling are the accessory movements. Three distinct types of accessory movements occur, known as *roll*, *slide* and *spin*.

Roll is similar to a car tyre rolling over the road surface. At any point, the same areas on the tyre will be in contact with the same areas on the road surface (*see* fig. 2.2(a)). If slide occurs, a single point on one surface will be in contact with a number of other points on the opposing surface, as when a car tyre skids (*see* fig 2.2(b)). Spin occurs when both points on the two opposing surfaces are in contact, and pure rotation occurs as with a 'spinning top' (*see* fig. 2.2(c)).

Accessory movements become important to general flexibility after injury. If a joint is stiff, stretching it will regain the physiological movements but may not bring back the accessory movements. This can leave the joint feeling awkward and open to injury. For this reason, it is always wise to see a physiotherapist after a sports injury to have the joint movement properly assessed.

Close and loose pack

The two opposing surfaces of a joint do not fit together exactly – they are said to be *noncongruent*. However, with the joint in one particular position its surfaces will come as close together as they are able, and this is known as 'close pack'. In this position the joint capsule and ligaments twist and pull the joint surfaces tightly together. The joint space is at a minimum, the concave surface of one bone fits closely on to the convex shape of the other, and no further movement is possible. In the close-pack position, stress will be taken on the bones in a fall because the ligaments in a joint are fully tightened and unable to 'give' any more. A fracture is often the result.

The loose-pack position is exactly the opposite. As the joint surfaces are released from their close-pack position, elastic recoil of

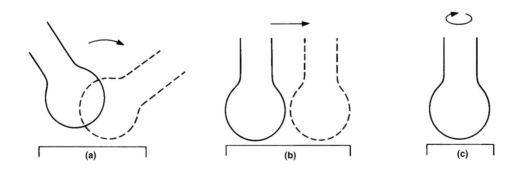

Figure 2.2 Accessory movements in a joint: (a) roll; (b) slide; (c) spin

the soft tissues surrounding the joint enables its surfaces to move apart, maximising the joint space. The joint will be less secure in this position and more movement will be possible. Should the athlete fall with the joint in a loose-pack position, the joint will often move too much, and ligament injury can result.

◆ Summary ◆

- There are over 200 bones in the body each made from calcium, phosphorous and proteins.
- Most bones begin life as cartilage and harden through a process of ossification.
- Synovial joints are surrounded by a capsule strengthened by ligaments.
- The joint contains synovial fluid, and the bone ends are covered by cartilage.
- Joints need regular movement to stay healthy.
- Joints have two types of movement: physiological and accessory.
- Physiological movements consist of bending, straightening and twisting, while accessory movements give the joint its healthy spring.
- In the close-pack position a joint is locked, in the loose-pack position it moves freely.

Chapter 3

Muscle Action

◆ How muscles work ◆

Muscle contraction itself is more important to strength training than to stretching. However, because stretching is primarily affecting muscle, it is vital that we have some understanding of the general principles underlying muscle actions.

Structure of a muscle

If we take a small piece of muscle tissue and magnify it many times (*see* fig. 3.1(a)), we can see that it is made up of many long muscle fibres. Each individual muscle fibre is surrounded by a thin membrane (endomysium), and in turn the fibres are grouped together in bundles covered by the *perimysium*. Finally, the whole muscle structure is encased in a sheath, the *epimysium*.

The muscle membranes stretch the whole length of the muscle from tendon to tendon, intimately linking the contractile and inert portions of the muscle. The whole structure is often referred to as the 'musculo-tendinous unit'. The combination of fibre contraction and elastic recoil of the mucle membranes is important for the development of 'elastic strength' (*see* page 28).

A further membrane, the *sarcolemma* surrounds the individual muscle cells. The sarcolemma is important because it is electrically conductive; it has within it, *sarcoplasm*, a

fluid containing fuel stores (glycogen) and enzymes important to muscle contraction. Within the sarcoplasm is an intricate membrane, the *sarcoplasmic reticulum*. This membrane contains transverse tubules, each of which end on the muscle cell surface as a lateral sac.

Looking closely at each fibre, we see alternating light and dark bands, corresponding to different muscle proteins. The light area is composed of a thin filament called *actin*, while the dark area consists of a thicker filament called *myosin*. The two sets of filaments fit together like the fingers on two opposing hands, one set of actin–myosin fibres being called a *sarcomere*. The thick myosin filament has projections or 'crossbridges' coming from it much like the oars of a boat. The thin actin filament has a long tropomyosin filament wound around it and a globular troponin molecule is positioned over this area. At rest the tropomyosin prevents (inhibits) actin and myosin from binding.

How do muscles contract?

Contraction of the muscle occurs when the muscle filaments move towards each other, and a whole sequence of events is required for this to take place. When we want a muscle to contract, a nervous impulse is sent from the brain. This impulse travels down the spinal cord and along a peripheral nerve to the muscle, where it causes changes on the

(a)

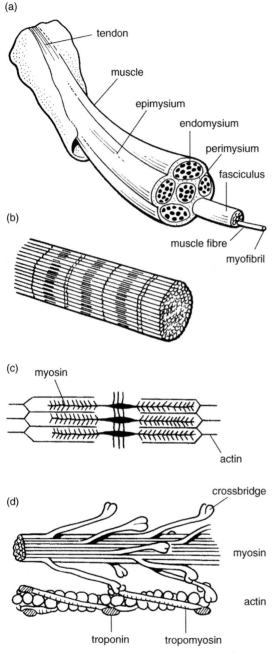

(b)

(c)

(d)

Figure 3.1(a) Structure of a muscle – contractile mechanism: (a) whole muscle and a group of muscle fibres; (b) a myofibril; (c) a sarcomere; (d) thick and thin filaments

surface of the muscle fibre. At the point where the nerve touches the muscle, a chemical (acetylcholine) is released which causes an electrical impulse to spread across the surface of the sarcolemma. As a result, calcium is released from the lateral sacs and passes down the transverse tubule to bind with the troponin molecule (*see* fig. 3.1(b)). This reaction causes the spiral trompomyosin to move deeper into the groove of the actin filament removing the inhibition. Once the inhibition has been removed, contraction will occur spontaneously, and the muscle filaments pull closer together causing them to slide over each other and shorten the muscle.

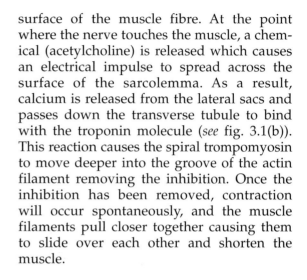

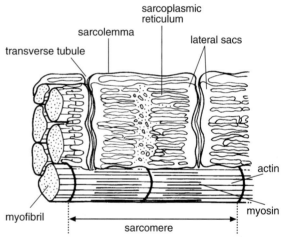

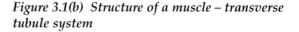

Figure 3.1(b) Structure of a muscle – transverse tubule system

The whole muscle contraction process uses energy, and rest is needed to recharge the structures involved. Calcium has to be moved out of the transverse tubule of the muscle and back into the lateral sacs. The filaments must then return to their original relaxed positions.

What affects muscle strength?

The amount of overlap that can occur between the sliding filaments of the muscle will determine its contractile strength, and the relationship between muscle length and tension development is called the length–tension relationship (*see* fig. 3.2). When the muscle is shortened, the filaments are over-lapped already and have little additional movement available to them. In the shortened position (inner range), therefore, the muscle is comparatively weak. In the lengthened position (outer range), the filaments have pulled apart and the actin and myosin elements are disengaged. Again the muscle is relatively 'weak' – it can produce little active force through contraction – however, because the muscle is now stretched, it is able to produce some force through elastic recoil. Therefore, the force in outer range is mostly created passively through recoil, rather than actively through contraction.

It is only in mid-range, when the muscle filaments are engaged but not overlapping, that maximal active force can be developed. Mid-range is the range that we use in our normal day-to-day activities, so functionally it is appropriate that this should be the strongest point in the available movement.

◆ Muscle reflexes ◆

Three muscle reflexes are important when using flexibility training: the *stretch reflex*; *autogenic inhibition* (also known as the reverse stretch reflex); and *reciprocal innervation*.

Stretch reflex

The *stretch reflex* is important both for postural control and muscle tone. It relies on information coming from special receptors called *muscle spindles* (*see* fig. 3.3(a)). The muscle spindle is a cigar-shaped structure attached alongside the main muscle fibres. When the muscle is stretched, so is the muscle spindle. The stretch of the spindle is detected by nerves and a reflex occurs that causes the muscle to contract and shorten the spindle once more.

The stretch reflex reacts to change in both the length of the muscle and in the velocity of its movement. Change in length is important for postural or *tonic* control, while change in velocity is important for movement or *phasic* control. The classic example of the stretch reflex acting for phasic control is the knee jerk, or patellar reflex. Here, the patella tendon is stretched rapidly by being hit with a small rubber hammer. This rapid stretch is picked up by the muscle spindles in the quadriceps and causes nerve impulses to be sent to the spinal cord. Impulses return from the cord to the quadriceps causing them to contract, and the knee straightens quickly giving a small 'kick'.

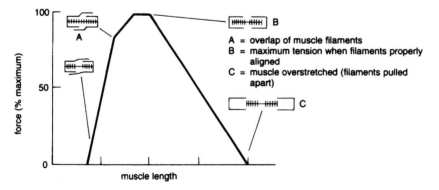

Figure 3.2 Length–tension relationship of a muscle

A = overlap of muscle filaments
B = maximum tension when filaments properly aligned
C = muscle overstretched (filaments pulled apart)

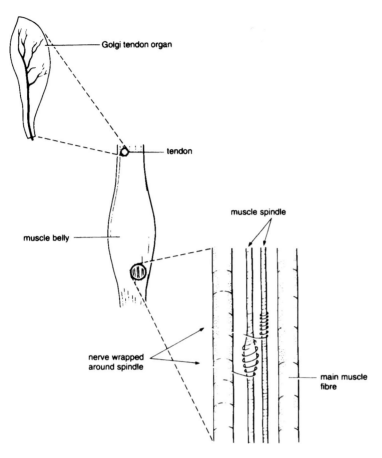

Figure 3.3(a) Muscle receptors

The third response (M3) occurs occasionally and is again a result of brain activity rather than the spinal cord. Voluntary contractions can occur within 170 ms of the detection of a movement, but the stretch reflex occurs much faster. M1 occurs within 30 ms and M2 within 50 to 60 ms. The stretch reflex therefore causes muscle contraction in response to an unexpected stretch some 140 ms (nearly one-fifth of a second) before voluntary muscle contraction.

The result is that the stretch initiates a contraction of the same muscle that limits the stretch itself, creating a negative feedback system sometimes referred to as a *resistance reflex*. The reflex is protective, tending to stabilise a joint and relies on a continuous barrage of nerve impulses coming from the joint itself. This process is known as *proprioception*.

After injury, these nerve impulses can be lessened (proprioception is impaired) tending to make a joint less stable. Therefore, an essential part of sports rehabilitation is the use of training to increase the number of nerve impulses being fed to a joint. This is achieved by performing a large variety of movements, especially those which tax balance skills, as these will feed more and more nerve impulses into the joint. This type of training, known as *proprioceptive exercise*, will help to restore the stability of a joint by improving the 'reaction time' of the muscles supporting it. In this way the stretch reflex is restored to its correct level of action and it is able once more to support the joint.

The stretch reflex is also essential for the maintenance of normal standing posture through tonic control. When we stand up we continually sway forwards and backwards. As we start to fall forwards there is a pull on our calf muscles, changing their length and causing a stretch reflex. The calf muscles then contract a split-second later to pull us back to the upright position again.

The reflex occurs in three parts (*see* fig. 3.3(b)). The first response is a short latency contraction (M1) that results from activation of the spinal reflex circuit itself. The second response is a long latency contraction (M2) that involves the lower centres of the brain.

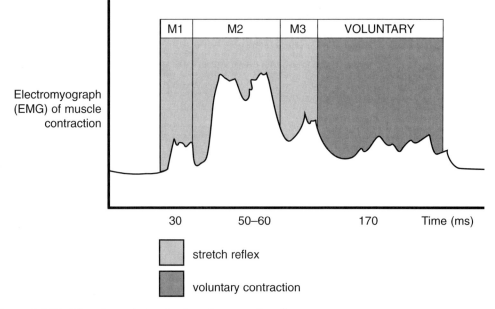

Figure 3.3(b) Muscle activity during the stretch reflex

Autogenic inhibition

Another receptor, the *golgi tendon organ* (GTO), is situated in the muscle tendon (*see* fig. 3.3(a)). This receptor measures tension. When a muscle contracts it shortens, so a stretch reflex will not occur. However, the GTO will register the increasing tension in the muscle tendon and will then cause a reflex relaxation of the muscle, a process known as *autogenic inhibition*. This is the reverse situation to the stretch reflex and has a protective function, preventing the muscle from contracting so hard that it pulls its attachment off the bone. The two reflexes do not occur at the same time, because the threshold of the GTO is set far higher than that of the muscle spindle. In normal everyday movement, tension in the muscle is not high enough to cause autogenic inhibition.

Both stretch and autogenic inhibition reflexes have important implications for stretching

exercises. Stretching which involves short jerking movements will tighten the muscle through the stretch reflex, while sustained stretching (over about 30 seconds) will allow the muscle to relax. Relaxation occurs because the stretch reflex becomes desensitised, and if the muscle tension is high enough autogenic inhibition follows through stimulation of the GTO. The autogenic inhibition in this case overrides the stretch reflex.

Reciprocal innervation

A further reflex is called *reciprocal innervation*. This occurs when the antagonist muscle relaxes to allow the prime mover to create a movement. For example, when the biceps muscle contracts to bend the elbow, the triceps will relax through reciprocal innervation to allow the movement to occur. This reflex can be used to obtain further relaxation in a muscle just prior to stretching.

◆ Elastic and contractile ◆ properties of muscle

Muscle has three properties: contractability, elasticity and extensibility.

Contractability

The contractile nature of muscle results from the movement of the sliding filaments within the muscle fibre.

Isometric
When the actin and myosin filaments come together, force is generated and the muscle will shorten. If the muscle filaments shorten, but the external length of the muscle remains the same, the muscle tenses but the joint on which the muscle works will not move. This is an *isometric* or static muscle contraction. An example is holding an object in the hand with the elbow bent to 90°.

Concentric
When the muscle filaments shorten and pull the attachments of the muscle closer to each other, causing movement at the joint, the muscle contraction is then *concentric*. In our example above, instead of the arm being held still, the elbow joint flexes. A concentric action tends to accelerate a limb. The movement begins slowly and gets faster.

Eccentric
Once the elbow has been flexed, and the muscle filaments shortened, lowering the weight again involves the muscle filaments slowly paying out to control the joint as it extends. This is an *eccentric* action. This type of action is used to slow the body down and control movements such as sitting down into a chair or coming downstairs. Each time, the muscle filaments are sliding apart and the muscle is lengthening.

Elasticity

Individual muscle fibres are grouped together in bundles (*see* page 23) and each fibre is surrounded by a connective tissue sheath (the endomysium). The bundles themselves are again aligned in groups and surrounded by another sheath (the epimysium). The muscle sheaths cannot contract, but they will stretch, and have important elastic properties. These elements of the muscle are known as the *parallel elastic components* because they are aligned parallel to the muscle fibres. The tendons at the end of the muscle are also non-contractile, but again they show elastic properties. These are the *series elastic components*, so called because they are positioned before and after the fibres.

We know that there is a linear relationship between load and elasticity from the load–deformation curve (*see* page 7). As we load a muscle it will stretch proportionally, and as the stretch ceases and the muscle springs back, energy is released.

Extensibility

If the stretch is applied slowly and released slowly, so that the muscle remains relaxed (non-contractile), the force produced by the muscle is purely passive. This is important in posture especially. As we bend forwards to touch our toes, the back muscles (erector spinae) are lengthening eccentrically to lower the trunk. However, these same muscles are also being placed on stretch. When we begin to come back up from the forward bend position, initially there is no muscle contraction. We begin our upward movement purely through elastic recoil of the back muscles, a process known as the *flexion relaxation response* (*see* fig. 3.3(c)). This mechanism is simply a way of conserving muscle energy, but it does illustrate the importance of maintaining

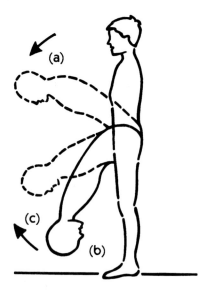

Figure 3.3(c) Flexion–relaxation response: (a) body is lowered by eccentric activity of the back muscles; (b) at full flexion the back muscles are fully stretched; (c) recoil of the stretched muscles begins the upward trunk movement: no muscle contraction is required initially

healthy elasticity within a muscle. For example, if a person suffers from chronic low back pain the flexion relaxation response no longer occurs because the back muscles are continuously in spasm and are unable to relax and stretch. The result is that the muscles have a poor blood flow (because blood no longer pumps through the muscle as it contracts and relaxes) and acids build up in the muscles causing pain.

As stretches become more rapid, the force produced is a combination of both elastic and contractile properties. When we lengthen a muscle its filaments move apart, ready to contract once more, and the elastic elements of the muscle are stretched. If this stretch is applied rapidly a stretch reflex occurs, causing the muscle to tighten and pull against the

stretching force. If the muscle contracts immediately afterwards, the contractile force produced will be a summation of contraction, elastic recoil, and reflex mechanisms and will be far greater than if the muscle contracted from rest (*see* fig. 3.4). This type of pre-stretching is used to advantage in plyometric training where a series of jumps and bounding movements are used to build up 'elastic strength'.

◆ Muscle fibres ◆

Types of muscle fibres

All muscles contain fibres of different types. Red fibres are designed to contract over and over again without fatiguing, and are known as *slow-twitch* fibres. White fibres are called *fast twitch*, and these give short bursts of power. A person's muscles will contain both fibre types but in different proportions. Those who are good at endurance sports tend to have more slow-twitch fibres in the leg muscles, while those who perform explosive sprints have more fast-twitch fibres (*see* fig. 3.5).

Arrangement of muscle fibres

No matter which type is present, each muscle fibre is only able to shorten and reduce its length by half. Although the same amount of shortening occurs with each fibre, altering the arrangement of these fibres within a muscle will affect muscle function. Two different arrangements are found, one for short powerful muscles and the other for long flexible ones.

The short powerful type is like the deltoid muscle of the shoulder. Here, the fibres are arranged side by side, inserting into a central tendon like the barbs on a feather. There are many of them so the muscle is very powerful.

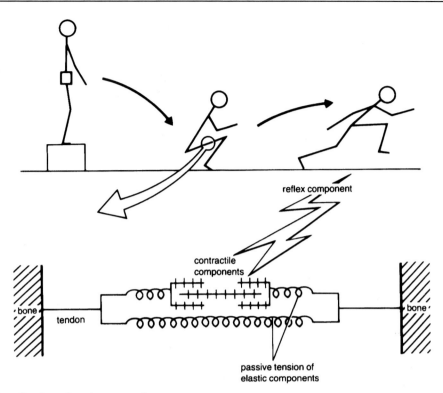

Figure 3.4 Developing elastic strength

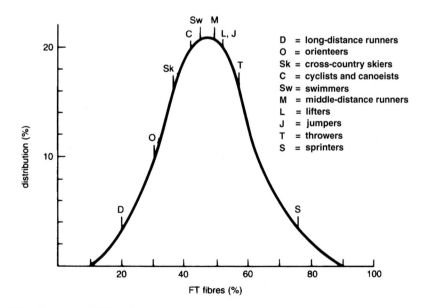

Figure 3.5 Distribution of fibre types

However, the fibres are short so the muscle cannot move very far and is therefore comparatively inflexible. This type of arrangement is called *pennate* (*see* fig. 3.6(a)).

Long slender muscles like the hamstrings on the back of the leg have their fibres arranged parallel to each other, attaching to tendons at each end (*see* fig. 3.6(b)). There are fewer fibres so the muscle is less powerful.

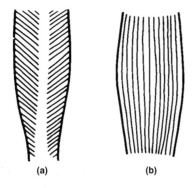

(a)   (b)

Figure 3.6 Arrangement of muscle fibres:
(a) shorter fibres of pennate muscle;
(b) longer fibres of parallel muscles

However, the muscle will still shorten by half, and as this type of muscle is much longer the movement it produces will be of a greater range. When choosing stretching exercises it is important to be aware of the underlying muscle structure to devise more effective programmes.

If we are throwing an object or hitting a ball we often need to develop the maximal amount of force possible. The amount of force will be dependent on our underlying strength, but also on the flexibility of a muscle and on the range of motion through which a limb is taken. This is because when we are able to use a greater range of motion we have more time to allow the speed of an object to build up. Take as an example the javelin throw. If an athlete has very stiff shoulders he or she will not be able to take the javelin very far back. An athlete with good flexibility around the shoulders will be able to develop greater force by accelerating the javelin for a longer period.

♦ Group action of muscles ♦

A muscle can only pull, it cannot decide which action to perform. We produce an infinite variety of actions with a finite number of muscles by combining the various actions in different ways. This co-ordinated action of the various muscles working on a body-part is called the *group action of muscles* (*see* table 3.1).

Prime mover (agonist)

When a muscle pulls to create a movement it is said to be acting as a *prime mover* or *agonist*. Most muscles can take on this function, depending on the action required and the site of the muscle. Other muscles may be able to help with the action, but are less effective than

Table 3.1 Group action of muscles (example: elbow flexion)

Prime mover (agonist)	Secondary (assistant) mover	Antagonist	Stabilisor (fixator)	Neutraliser
Creates primary movement (*biceps*)	Assists prime mover (*brachialis*)	If contracted, would oppose prime mover (*triceps*)	Stabilises or fixes bone origin of prime mover (*shoulder muscles*)	Removes unwanted action of prime mover (*pronators*)

the prime mover. The muscles which help are called *secondary* or *assistant movers*. If we take elbow flexion as an example, both biceps and brachialis can flex the elbow. In most circumstances the biceps is more effective and so acts as the prime mover, the brachialis as the secondary mover.

Antagonist

The muscle that would oppose the prime mover if it is contracted is known as the *antagonist*. If we bend the arm the biceps will act as the prime mover to create the power necessary to carry out the movement. To allow the movement to occur, however, the opposite muscle – in this case the triceps – must relax and in so doing acts as an antagonist (*see* fig. 3.7).

Stabilisor (fixator)

Muscles do not simply create movements; they are also able to stabilise parts of the body or prevent unwanted actions by acting as *stabilisors* or *fixators*. In this case the muscle will contract to steady or support the bone on to which the prime mover attaches. Take as an example the sit-up exercise. The abdominal muscles attach from the rib-cage to the pelvis, so when they contract they will move both body areas, tending to posteriorly tilt the pelvis and pull the rib-cage down. To allow the abdominals to contract more effectively we need to fix one body area to provide a firm base for the muscles to pull on. This occurs by the hip flexor muscles acting as fixators to stop the pelvis from tilting as the abdominals contract. In the case of elbow flexion, mentioned above, because the biceps attach to the shoulder girdle, these bones must be stabilised to stop them sliding on the rib-cage as the biceps contracts.

Neutraliser

Many muscles can perform more than one movement. In the case of the biceps, for example, as well as flexing the elbow the muscle can also twist the forearm upwards (supination). If we want the biceps to perform just one action, bending the arm but not twisting it, other muscles must contract to stop the biceps from twisting the forearm. These muscles, which eliminate unwanted actions, are acting as *neutralisers*. As we saw above, the biceps muscle cannot decide which action to perform and which not to perform. Again it must be emphasised that a muscle can only pull: if we want to alter the action it will produce we must bring other muscles into play as neutralisers.

♦ Two-joint muscles ♦

Some muscles cross over two joints, and are said to be *biarticular*. The hamstrings, for example, attach from the seat bone (ischial tuberosity) to the top of the tibia. Because they cross both the hip and knee joints they are capable of creating, or limiting, movement at both joints. Other muscles which are biarticular include the rectus femoris and gastrocnemius in the lower limbs, and the biceps and triceps in the upper limbs. Biarticular muscles have a number of important biomechanical features.

Passive insufficiency

First, because they pass over two joints, they cannot shorten enough to allow full movement at both joints simultaneously. For example, with the knee bent and the hamstrings relaxed at the knee, the hip can flex maximally enabling the knee to be pulled right up

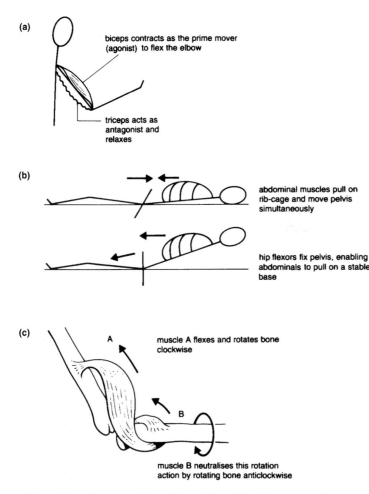

(a)

biceps contracts as the prime mover
(agonist) to flex the elbow

triceps acts as
antagonist and
relaxes

(b)

abdominal muscles pull on
rib-cage and move pelvis
simultaneously

hip flexors fix pelvis, enabling
abdominals to pull on a stable
base

(c)

A

muscle A flexes and rotates bone
clockwise

B

muscle B neutralises this rotation
action by rotating bone anticlockwise

Figure 3.7 Group action of muscles: (a) prime mover/
antagonist; (b) fixator; (c) neutraliser

into extension first, however, and try the same movement, you will find that you are unable to touch your heel to your buttock. This is because in the first example the upper portion of the hamstrings was lengthened and the lower part shortened. In the second example, the upper and lower parts of the muscle are unable to shorten fully at the same time. This inability to create full movement at both joints simultaneously is called *active insufficiency*.

Concurrent movement

Because biarticular muscles are unable to permit full movement at both joints at the same time, the tension in one muscle will cause tension to build up in its antagonist. For example, if the hamstrings contract and extend the hip they will stretch the rectus femoris which is acting as an antagonist. The stretch in the rectus will then tend to pull the knee straight and extend it. When both the hip and knee are extending in this fashion, *concurrent movement* is said to be occurring. If we look at what happens to the muscle we can see that this type of action actually conserves energy. The hip and knee are both extending, so the hamstrings are shortened at their upper end and lengthened at their lower end. The rectus femoris is shortened at its lower end and lengthened higher up. This action has therefore avoided both active and passive insufficiency, by neither shortening nor stretching both ends of either muscle. It is used in running as we push off from the ground.

on to the chest (*see* fig. 3.8). However, with the knee straight, and the lower portion of the hamstrings stretched, hip flexion is more limited. This limitation of movement at both joints is called *passive insufficiency*.

Active insufficiency

If you stand up and flex your hip you will be able to bend your knee actively to touch your buttock with your heel. If you pull your hip

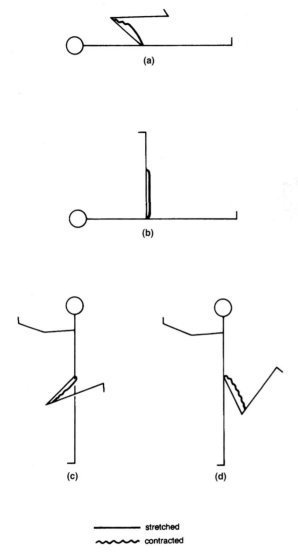

stretched
contracted

Figure 3.8 Active and passive insufficiency of a muscle: (a) hamstrings stretched at hip but relaxed at the knee; (b) hamstrings stretched over both joints (passive insufficiency); (c) hamstring stretched at the hip and contracted at the knee; (d) hamstrings contracted at both joints (active insufficiency)

Countercurrent movement

In a kicking action the opposite occurs. When the hip is flexed and the knee extended both the upper and lower portions of the rectus femoris are shortened, while both parts of the hamstrings are lengthened. The rectus therefore rapidly loses tension while the hamstrings rapidly gain tension, an example of *countercurrent movement*.

♦ Muscle imbalance and ♦ core stability

Muscles can be broadly categorised into two types, depending on how they function in day-to-day activities (*see* table 3.2). Some muscles, for example gluteals, act as postural or *stabilising* muscles, while others, for example hamstrings, act as locomotion or *movement* muscles.

Table 3.2 Muscle imbalance

Stabilising muscles (postural)	Movement muscles (locomotion)
Characteristics	**Characteristics**
Deep	Superficial
Predominently slow-twitch	Predominently fast-twitch
Single joint	Two-joint
Reduced activity (inhibited)	Preferential recruitment
Lengthen	Tighten
Light resistance	High resistance and ballistic
Correction	**Correction**
Improve tone and endurance	Stretch the tight muscles

Stabilising muscles

Stabilising muscles tend to be placed deeply within the body and act as postural muscles. Examples would include the deep abdominals (transversus abdominis) and the deep spinal muscles (multifidus), as well as the gluteals in many situations (*see* table 3.3). These muscles are built for endurance and have many slow-twitch fibres. They contract minimally, but hold the contraction for a long time. Unfortunately, in a person with an inactive lifestyle, or in someone who is active but has poor alignment, the stabilising muscles often have very poor tone and tend to sag. They almost seem to 'give way to gravity'. The tone is poor in these muscles not because they are weak, but because the nerve impulses, which control all muscles, find it difficult to get through to the muscle, and we say that the muscle has *poor recruitment*.

Table 3.3 Examples of muscle types

Stabilising muscles	Movement muscles
Deep abdominals	Superficial abdominals
Gluteals	Hamstrings
Vastus medialis	Rectus femoris
Soleus	Gastrocnemius
Serratus anterior	Pectoralis major
Lower trapezius	Latissimus dorsi

The poor recruitment of the muscle occurs because the muscles have been infrequently used, and often because a person has had pain. For example, when a person has knee pain one of the stabilising muscles of the knee (vastus medialis) will waste, and the same is true of other regions of the body. When we have back pain, our deep abdominals and our deep spinal muscles tend to waste and the nerve impulses to these muscles are reduced.

Because the muscles have not been used, we find it difficult to switch them back on – it is a case of 'use it or loose it'.

Movement muscles

Movement muscles, on the other hand, tend to be more superficial, for example the hamstrings on the back of the thigh and rectus femoris on the front. These muscles are very active in sport, being our sprinting and kicking muscles. They work over two joints, in this case the knee and hip, and tend to get very tight and powerful as they are recruited by hard and fast exercise and heavy poundages such as in weight training.

Correcting the imbalance

Because many forms of training tend to involve harder and faster movements, i.e. go for the burn, rather than slow controlled actions, for example yoga and tai chi, we end up with an imbalance of muscle length and tension around a joint. The imbalance leaves us with tight, strong superficial muscles on the one hand and sagging, poorly toned, deeper postural muscles. This gives rise to a number of postural problems and leaves us open to muscle injury through tearing. To correct the imbalance we must do three things: stretch the tight muscles; improve the tone and endurance of the postural muscles by shortening them; and correct any alignment problems which have occurred (*see* Chapter 5).

To begin with we must work for core stability. This involves tightening the abdominal muscles (*see* page 61) to provide a stable base before we begin stretching. If we fail to do this, as we stretch our alignment may be very poor. In figure 3.9 the subject is trying to stretch the rectus femoris muscle on the front

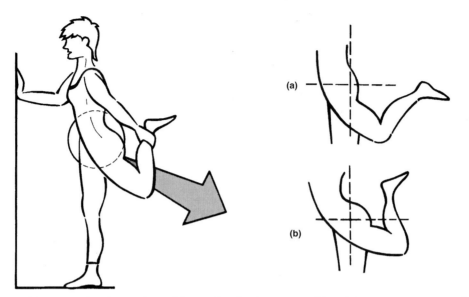

Figure 3.9 (a) Normal pelvic tilt and lower back alignment; (b) pelvis moves excessively, causing lower back to hollow; leg goes higher, but technique is faulty

of the thigh by flexing the knee and extending the hip at the same time. To do this, **the pelvis must remain stable**, and must not move. However, in this diagram the subject has been unable to hold the abdominal muscles tight enough to stop the pelvis from tilting forwards. They are unable to *stabilise* the lumbo-pelvic region. The stress from this exercise is therefore thrown on to the lower back potentially causing back injury. For this reason, learning to stabilise the lumbo-pelvic region is essential before lower limb stretching exercises begin. This technique is described on pages 60–2.

♦ Summary ♦

- A muscle is made up of actin and myosin filaments, which slide together causing the muscle to contract.
- There are three muscle reflexes relevant to stretching: the stretch reflex, autogenic inhibition, and reciprocal innervation.
- Muscle demonstrates contractability (pull), extensibility (stretch) and elasticity (spring).
- Muscles consist of slow-twitch fibres built for endurance and fast-twitch fibres built for power.
- A muscle that creates a movement is a prime mover (agonist); the muscle that relaxes to allow a movement to occur is the antagonist.
- A muscle may also hold a body-part firm (stabiliser) or prevent an unwanted secondary action (neutraliser).
- A biarticular muscle works over two joints.
- Stabilising muscles tend to become lax and sag; movement muscles tighten.

Chapter 4

Principles of Training

◆ Warm-up ◆

Before starting any exercise session, it is essential to warm up. There are two main reasons for this: first, warming-up can make sports injuries less likely in certain circumstances; second, the body works more efficiently when warm and sports performance may actually improve. A good warm-up will have physiological, mechanical and psychological effects.

Physiological effects

It takes some time for the body to change from its basic 'tick over' at rest to a point at which it is ready to perform maximally. If vigorous exercise is started immediately from rest, the heartbeat is speeded up with a jolt instead of increasing gradually, and the beats of the heart can become irregular, rather than showing their normal smooth rhythm. These changes affecting the heart can be potentially very serious in the older or less active individual, and especially in those with a history of heart or circulatory problems.

Effects on the heart
In 1973 an important study was conducted which showed the importance of warm-up to the cardio-vascular system (Barnard et al. 1973). Researchers took a group of men with no history of heart problems and made them run vigorously on a treadmill for 10–15 seconds without a warm-up. In 70% of these subjects, abnormal changes were seen on an electrocardiogram (ECG) machine. These changes, called *ischaemia* showed that insufficient blood was getting to the heart muscle, a potentially very dangerous situation. However, when the same subjects ran on the treadmill after performing a warm-up, the ECG changes were greatly reduced, and in many cases the trace was completely normal, demonstrating considerably less strain being imposed on the heart. In addition, blood pressure (BP) was taken when the subjects ran on the treadmill both with and without a warm-up. Average blood pressures of 168 mmHg were taken in those subjects who ran without a warm-up, while for those who did a warm-up, the blood pressure averaged 140 mmHg, some 12% lower. Again, these changes demonstrated the importance of a warm-up in reducing the strain placed on the heart by vigorous exercise.

Effect on body tissue
A warm-up will allow the body tissues to work more efficiently. Normally, while relaxed, the muscles receive only about 15% of the total blood flow. The rest goes to the body organs such as the brain, liver and intestines. During vigorous exercise, because the muscles need far more fuel to provide energy, their requirement for blood increases and they need 80% of the total blood flow. It takes time to re-route this blood by opening

some blood vessels and closing others, and if the muscles are required to perform maximally before the blood flow has changed they will work inefficiently.

Incidentally, this process of alteration in regional blood flow is the reason why you should not exercise within an hour of eating a heavy meal. After eating, we need the blood to stay in the region of the stomach and intestines to effectively absorb the digested foodstuffs. If we start to exercise during this period, much of the blood will move away from the digestive organs and into the working muscles. The result can be digestive upsets and 'stomach cramps'.

Lactic acid formation

The body can produce energy by two methods: aerobically (with oxygen) and anaerobically (without oxygen). The aerobic method is preferable, because when we work anaerobically we produce a waste product called lactic acid. Unfortunately, we cannot work aerobically straightaway as it takes time to switch the aerobic system on. If we start intense exercise without a warm-up, the aerobic system does not have enough time to switch on; we therefore have to provide energy anaerobically, with resultant lactic acid formation.

The function of a warm-up is to 'switch on' the aerobic system and allow the body to reach a steady state where the energy provided by the body exactly matches its requirements through exercise. Once this is done, less waste is produced and so our recovery after exercise will be much faster.

Mechanical effects

The mechanical effects of warm-up occur as a direct result of tissue heating. Chemical reactions involved in the production of energy for the working muscle and the removal of waste

products are speeded up with warmth. In addition, nerve impulses travel faster when a nerve is warm. The effects of a warm-up on nerve conduction is particularly important for the speed of reflexes, which protect the muscles from injury.

When a substance is heated it becomes more pliable, and this is exactly the same for the body tissues. We have seen that there is a relationship between load and deformation of a tissue (*see* fig. 1.8). One of the effects of warm-up is to move the load–deformation curve to the right. This means that, for any given load, a warm tissue will be elastic for longer and will reach its failure point later. The effect of these changes is to make stretching exercises both more effective and safer. In addition, the fluid within a joint becomes less stiff (viscous) when warm so the joint will move more smoothly.

Figure 4.1 shows the effect of heat on a tendon as it is stretched. Because tissues will stretch more easily after a warm-up, it is important that stretching exercises are not performed at the beginning of a warm-up period. Vigorously touching the toes will not act as a warm-up for the hamstrings, and may tear them instead!

Psychological effects

Two effects are important here: arousal level and mental rehearsal.

Arousal level

There is a direct relationship between arousal and performance, and this can be illustrated on the *human performance curve* (*see* fig. 4.2). Initially, as arousal increases so does performance. However, after a certain point an individual becomes too aroused (they are now 'stressed') and their performance suffers. As an illustration of this mechanism, imagine you have had a boring day and you arrive at

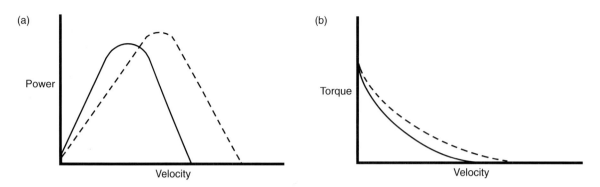

Figure 4.1 Vertical jump test: effect of tissue temperature increase due to a warm-up: (a) peak power increases, demonstrated by the increased height; (b) maximum velocity of shortening increases, and torque–velocity curve shifts to the right. After Enoka, 1994

the gym not really wanting to exercise. Your arousal level is low so your exercise performance will be poor. If you then go into an exercise class, however, the instructor, the music and the other people, will increase your arousal level. You feel motivated and your exercise performance improves. On the other hand, imagine if you are an athlete competing in an important game and you miss a shot that normally you would find very easy. Perhaps you are nervous, your heart is pounding and your arousal level is too high, so your performance suffers.

The function of a warm-up should be to place an individual at the optimum point on the human performance curve; this will change depending on the individual and the sport. A person who is very introverted and under-aroused may need to be 'psyched up' in a warm-up to move them to the right on the curve. Someone who is aggressive, extrovert and 'hyperactive' may need to be calmed down and moved further to the left on the curve. Events which require highly skilled movements tend to be performed better at lower levels of arousal when an individual is calm and can focus his or her attention. Events which require power or explosive actions are normally performed better when higher levels of arousal are achieved. This is why stretching exercises are best performed after a gentle but thorough warm-up to heat the body tissues, but relax the mind.

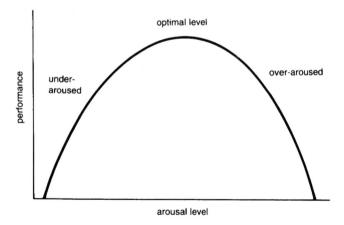

Figure 4.2 Human performance curve

Mental rehearsal

The second psychological effect of a warm-up is that of mental rehearsal. Complex actions tend to be forgotten between exercise bouts. The first or second repetition of a complex action may not be as good as the fourth or fifth, when you have had time to 'get into' the movement. With skilled actions it is essential that we rehearse the movement, slowly going through a golf swing, for example, before we perform the action at full speed. This is very important with activities, such as dance and martial arts, that require a high degree of active flexibility.

Types of warm-up

A warm-up can either be 'passive', with the body heated from the outside, or 'active', using exercise to form the heat internally. An example of a passive warm-up is to have a sauna or hot shower. An active warm-up can be achieved through gentle jogging or using light aerobics. Both types can be effective, but are appropriate in different situations.

An active warm-up is the type normally used before exercise, while the passive warm-up is useful when stretching a muscle tightened from a previous strain. The advantage of the passive warm-up, from the point of view of injury, is that it does not require the athlete to move the injured tissues in order to create body-heat. The use of external heat can also reduce pain and muscle spasm, helping the muscle to relax and allowing the stretch to be taken further.

In addition to active and passive types, a warm-up may also be either general or specific. A general warm-up, such as jogging or static cycling, will affect the whole body. The effects here are mainly on the major body systems such as the heart, lungs and blood vessels. This should be followed by a specific warm-up which concentrates on the body-part and action to be used in a particular exercise. The effects now are more localised, mainly affecting body tissues used in the actual exercise and rehearsing the action to be performed.

Warm-up techniques

The amount of exercise required for an effective warm-up will depend very much on a person's fitness level and the exercise to be performed in the main part of the workout. This is because changes in body temperature vary with body-size, fat level and rate of body metabolism. In addition, sports differ tremendously in the demand they make on the body tissues, so a warm-up before a vigorous game of hockey would clearly need to be more extensive than one for a casual game of bowls. Equally, a top level sprinter will require a more thorough warm-up session than a casual sportsman or woman, because the sprinter is likely to be able to push him or herself to a higher physical level. The following are general guidelines.

- **Intensity**: If it is to be effective, a warm-up must be intense enough to cause mild sweating. When this happens it indicates that the inside (core) temperature of the body has increased by about 1°C. Increasing the core temperature by this amount has been shown to be the minimum requirement for bringing about the warm-up changes discussed above.

- **Clothing**: Because we are trying to raise the body temperature, it is best to perform the warm-up wearing warm clothing to keep the body-heat in. The amount of clothing needed to provide adequate insulation will depend largely on the outside temperature. Light clothing may be suitable in a warm sports-hall, but thick fleecy material with a weatherproof covering layer will be needed on the touch-line of a cold and windy pitch.

- **Activities**: Warm-up activities should be continuous and rhythmical in nature. Gentle jogging, light aerobics, or cycling on a static bicycle in the gym are all examples of good warm-up activities. Once light sweating has begun, the major joints should be taken through their full range of movement, starting with small movements which gradually become larger. Finally, some sport-specific actions must be included in the warm-up period as a part of skill rehearsal.

- **Time**: A good warm-up may take 10–15 minutes, but it is time well spent. Note that we are using a warm-up before stretching rather than using stretching as part of a warm-up. This makes sense because tissues will stretch more effectively when warm. The movements we use in the warm-up to take the major joints through their range of motion are not stretching exercises as such. The warm-up movements take the joints through their full range of motion, but do not try to increase this range of motion as stretching exercises would.

♦ Warm-down ♦

Just as it is vital to begin an exercise session slowly by warming up, so it is important to end it the same way by using a warm-down or cool-down. The warm-down period has a number of important effects.

First, during intense exercise the heartbeat increases, and the beating of the heart is actually helped by the contraction of the exercising limb muscles. As these muscles contract they squeeze the blood vessels which travel through them, thus helping the blood to return to the heart. If an individual stops exercising suddenly, the limb muscles no longer pump the blood vessels and help the heart. The demand placed on the heart is increased and the pulse will actually get faster although exercise has stopped.

An effective warm-down can also reduce muscle ache. This is caused partly by lactic acid formation, and partly through tiny muscle tears which occur during very hard training. Hard training causes local swelling within a muscle, giving *delayed onset muscle soreness* (DOMS). In the case of DOMS, you feel fine the day after a workout, but the day after that you feel stiff. To reduce these effects you should perform a warm-down using similar exercises to those chosen for the warm-up, gradually lowering the exercise intensity until resting levels are reached. It is interesting to note that stretching exercises may be used to reduce muscle pain that occurs after intensive strength training.

Finally, shake your muscles to loosen and relax them, and take a warm shower to flush fresh blood through them and aid recovery. Because blood is still needed in the muscles after exercise in order to aid recovery, you should not eat a large meal immediately. If you feel hungry and in need of an 'energy boost' eat a small amount of sweet, high-carbohydrate food such as a banana or a piece of toast and honey.

♦ Overload ♦

To achieve a training effect, the body must be exposed to a physical stress which is greater than that encountered in everyday living. If this is done the body is said to be *overloaded*, and the body tissues will change or 'adapt' as a result, provided they are given time to do so. The two key points regarding overload are: that the overload must be greater than that normally encountered by the body; and that time is needed for the body tissues to adapt. Tissue adaptation of this type can be illustrated by something rubbing on the skin, such as a stone in a shoe. If the rubbing occurs continuously (without rest), the skin will break down and bleed. If, however, the rubbing occurs and then the skin is rested before being stressed again, a hard callus will form. In the former case, no recovery period was available for tissue adaptation, in the latter, tissue adaptation (callus growth) occurred in the recovery period itself. Exactly the same occurs with exercise.

If we take weight training as an example of this process, the resistance from the weight causes muscle breakdown. The body overcompensates by building stronger muscle in the rest period between exercise. For this reason, rest is vital, and intense exercise should not be practised every day, but on alternate days.

As fitness improves, exercise must become harder so the body continues to be taxed to the same degree. If the body has adapted to the training load, further improvement will only occur if the training intensity is increased. Exercise must therefore be progressive (gradually getting harder) for the overload to have the same effect.

Overload has four components: type, intensity, duration, and frequency (*see* table 4.1).

- **Type**: The training type will dictate the tissue changes which will occur, and the training is said to be 'specific'. For each of the components of fitness (*see* table 4.2) a different training type is required. When training for stamina the intensity of exercise may be determined by the pulse rate, and when training for strength by the weight lifted.

- **Intensity and duration**: Training must be intense enough to challenge the body tissues, and of sufficient duration for the challenge to continue long enough. The

intensity of flexibility training may be assessed by the range of movement and how long the stretch is held.

- **Frequency**: The frequency must be appropriate – often enough for the tissues changes to build up, but not too often so that recovery is allowed.

Table 4.2 Fitness components ('S' factor)

Stamina	Cardiopulmonary and local muscle endurance
Suppleness	Active, passive, PNF
Strength	Concentric, eccentric, isometric
Speed	Speed (rate of movement), power (rate of doing work
Skill	Balance and co-ordination
Specificity	Exercise must match required training outcome
Spirit	Psychological factors of training

The American College of Sports Medicine (ACSM) defined the appropriate overload for health-related exercise in 1978, and this was updated in 1990. They say that the quality and quantity of exercise required to maintain aerobic fitness and body composition is a training frequency of three to five days per week at an intensity of between 60–90% of the age-related maximal heart rate. This should

Table 4.1 Overload components

Type	*Intensity*	*Duration*	*Frequency*
Fitness component ('S' factor)	How hard	How long	How often

be carried out for 20–60 minutes each time and be rhythical or continuous in nature. Resistance training should be performed for one set of 8–12 repetitions of 8–10 exercises for the major muscle groups for two days per week.

No recommendation is given for stretching exercise quality and quantity, but the following are some general recommendations.

- Stretch the major joints and two-joint muscles 3–5 times per week.

- Hold each stretch for 20–30 seconds.

- Stretch after a warm-up of sufficient intensity to induce light sweating.

◆ Training effects ◆

We have seen that an overload on body tissue gives a training effect. This effect is largely reversible, however. If training stops, the benefits achieved for each fitness component will be lost and 'detraining' will occur.

In just 20 days of total rest, stamina reduces by 25% – a loss of about 1% per day. Strength reduction is even greater, with average losses over the same period of 35%. Muscles that have become more flexible with training will slowly tighten again, and muscle imbalance may occur if some muscles tighten more quickly than others (*see* page 33). Skill-based components including sports technique, balance and co-ordination last longer, but will gradually degrade with time. The principle is clear – 'use it or lose it!'

Training has immediate, short-term and long-term effects.

- **Immediate** effects are the body's responses to exercise. These are brought about by increased metabolism and include higher heart and breathing rates, changes in blood flow, increased body temperature, and chemical alterations to enzymes within the working muscles.

- **Short-term** training effects become apparent when exercise stops and the body tries to reduce its metabolic rate to resting levels once more. Body temperature has increased, so sweating continues to try to cool the tissues. Energy has been used and must be replaced, so breathing rate and heart rate remain high. Waste products have been formed as energy was 'burnt', and these wastes must be eliminated.

- **Long-term** effects are the cumulative results of exercise, reflecting the body's adaptation to training. Intense training stresses the body; over time, the body learns from this and changes so that the next training bout will not stress it as much. If a training session is not intense enough, it will not stress the body sufficiently and no adaptation will occur. However, if it is too intense and the body cannot cope, injury may result. Following training, time must be allowed for the body to change and adapt, so rest for recovery from exercise is vital.

◆ Components of fitness ◆

It is generally accepted that two types of fitness exist: health-related and task- (performance) related. These include various components which can be described as 'S' factors for convenience (*see* table 4.2). Health-related fitness includes components that are considered to be beneficial to health. In this context the term *stamina* is used to encompass both heart–lung fitness and muscle endurance. This fitness component is important to the health of the heart and circulatory system. *Suppleness* (flexibility) and *strength* are concerned with the health of the musculo-skeletal system, and are important in injury prevention.

These three components are all essential to sports performance, but in addition *speed* and *skilled action* are required. Speed involves rapid muscle contraction and the elastic abilities of the muscle (*see* page 28) and is important for explosive events. Skill includes the skills needed for a particular sport, as well as general skills such as balance and co-ordination.

Injury will be more likely if the fitness components become unbalanced. For example, an inexperienced bodybuilder may have excessive strength in comparison with their flexibility, making muscle pulls more likely. A poorly trained distance runner may have a lot of stamina to protect the heart, but very little strength or flexibility, leaving the joints open to injury. Many keep-fit enthusiasts see themselves as 'very fit' because they may be strong and supple and have plenty of stamina; but endless hours spent working on gym machines will do little to improve skill, and fitness enthusiasts can be left clumsy with poor balance and co-ordination ability. So the message is clear: an overall training programme must work on **all** the fitness components if it is to be totally effective.

◆ Specificity ◆

Over a period of time, the demands placed on the body during exercise cause the body to change. With stretching, the muscles become more flexible; with weight training they become stronger; and with running, stamina improves. These changes are the adaptations to exercise and will closely match the type of demand placed on the body. For example, running marathons will improve aerobic endurance, while sprinting will build anaerobic power. If we wanted to improve our distance-running ability there would be little point in using sprint training, because the body adaptation that would occur would not be the right one.

SAID principle

The above example illustrates an important principle, that of *training specificity*. We can say that all training follows the SAID principle: 'specific adaptation to imposed demand'. Put simply, this dictates that the change which takes place in the body (the adaptation) will closely resemble (be specific to) the type of training used (the imposed demand).

Applying this principle to stretching means that when choosing stretching exercises to improve sports performance we must match the range of motion, the muscles stretched, and the muscle balance around a joint to similar actions in the desired sport. For example, if a soccer player needs stretching exercises, these can be designed for the muscles used in kicking. The exercises should take account of any tightness a player may already have, and the stretching programme should be individually designed. Also, stretching should be applied as part of a general training programme, so that increases in flexibility are matched by strength improvements, which enable the player to control the new range of motion which he or she has gained.

◆ Flexibility training ◆

What stops a joint moving through an infinite range of motion?

We need to look at two areas to explain this: internal (body) factors and external (environmental) factors.

One important internal factor is bone. Obviously we cannot affect the amount of bone in a joint, but we must be aware of it as a limiting factor to flexibility. After a fracture, for example, the amount of bone will increase over the fracture site. If this area is near a joint, range of motion may be reduced: in this case it would be fruitless to continue a stretching programme to this region. Equally, an elderly athlete may have osteoarthrosis, a condition in which the bone surfaces of the joints become uneven and more bone is formed. Again, the bone itself may limit movement and it would be dangerous to attempt any forceful stretching manoeuvres. Soft tissues such as tendons, ligaments, the joint capsule and the skin itself will limit movement. These tissues are *inert*, i.e. they do not contract. However, they do have elastic properties so they will stretch. Muscle is also an important factor: it is contractile and its contraction is governed by a number of important reflexes. Surrounding the muscle, however, is a connective tissue framework which will limit movement, so a muscle may be seen as both an inert and contractile structure.

The most important external factor that affects flexibility is temperature. When warmed, the body tissues become more pliable. A thorough warm-up must, therefore, be performed before stretching exercises are attempted. Often, vigorous stretching exercises are performed as a warm-up, which is incorrect: until the tissues are warm, and an athlete starts to sweat lightly, full-range stretching exercises should not be attempted. In the same way that warm tissue is more pliable, cold tissue is stiffer. Research has shown that when stretching is used after injury a greater range of motion can be achieved if the muscle is cooled with ice while holding it in its final stretched position.

Individual differences in flexibility

If you ask the members of any class to perform a stretching exercise you immediately see a tremendous variation in movement: some will be more flexible than others; some will move into the position in a smooth and effortless way; while others will stumble clumsily into the exercise. The differences reflect variations in both range of movement and skill-level between individuals.

Individuals involved in strength and power events are usually less flexible than those who use their own body-weight as resistance, such as swimmers, gymnasts, and dancers. The degree of flexibility depends also on whether a person's fitness programme is balanced. Inexperienced bodybuilders who just train for strength and bulk are among the least flexible, while teenage girl gymnasts can be among the most flexible.

Females are generally more flexible than males, especially around the hip and shoulder. Hormonal changes will also affect flexibility in females. During pregnancy, and to a lesser extent during menstruation, *relaxin* hormone is released into the bloodstream. This, together with progesterone and oestrogen, has the effect of relaxing the pelvic ligaments, and making the joint between the base of the spine and the pelvis (the sacroiliac joint) more mobile. The effects of hormone changes may remain for as long as six months after pregnancy, so during this time the individual is at risk from rapid end-range stretching exercises.

Range of movement is also dictated by lifestyle and previous injury. Inactive individuals who get the exercise message late in life will be inflexible, and in many cases the range of movement they gain will never be as great as the range they could have achieved, had they been active all their lives. In addition, the limitation to range of movement can often be permanent, dictated by years of poor posture and faulty movement techniques. Previous injuries can leave a reduced range of movement as the only outward sign that problems have occurred. Individuals with a history of low back pain will often be tight in the lower spine and hamstring muscles, while those with shoulder problems may be left with limited shoulder rotation movements. In cases where an individual's flexibility is asymmetrical (greater on one side of the body than the other), a flexibility programme must aim to restore symmetry and not just increase range of movement.

Flexibility and body type

Each of us has a different type of body: some are fatter, some are thinner, and some are more or less muscled. The degree to which we differ can be partially explained by our 'body type' or *somatotype*. Three extreme body types are recognised: *mesomorphs* (muscular); *endomorphs* (fatter); and *ectomorphs* (thinner) (*see* fig. 4.3).

- **Mesomorphs** have more bone and muscle development. Their bodies are made for strenuous physical activity, and individuals of this type tend to be heavily muscled. The chest is broad, and the shoulders are wider than the waist – the 'Tarzan' type.

- **Endomorphs** have rounder physiques and they tend to put on and store fat. They have a 'pear drop' appearance with the abdomen

being as large or larger than the chest – the typical 'Billy Bunter' character.

- **Ectomorphs** have long delicate limbs – the traditional 'bean-poles'.

In reality, few people have physiques which fall firmly into just one of these categories. We are all a mixture of the three extremes. By taking height, weight, bone size, limb girth and body-fat measurements, an individual can be given a score indicating the proportion of each body-type component present in their physiques.

Scores range from 1 to 7, and are presented in the order endomorph/mesomorph/ectomorph. Thus a highly endomorphic individual would score 7/1/1 and a high mesomorph 1/7/1. The somatotype rating can be illustrated graphically so that somatotype averages for different sports can be compared (*see* fig. 4.4). We can see, for example, that both gymnasts and basketball players have a high degree of mesomorphy, but that the basketball players have a greater tendency to endomorphy than do the gymnasts. Body-builders are highly mesomorphic, as we

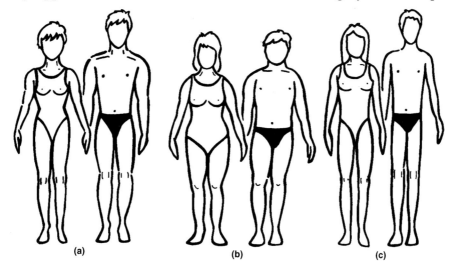

Figure 4.3 Somatotypes – the three extremes of body types: (a) mesomorph; (b) endomorph; (c) ectomorph

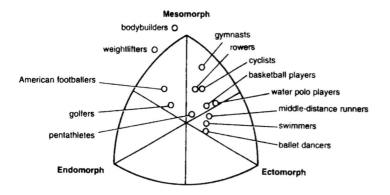

Figure 4.4 Elite athlete somatotypes

would expect. Both ballet dancers and swimmers are roughly average on all scores, possibly reflecting the fact that these athletes use their own body-weight as resistance.

Flexibility methods

We have seen that range of motion can be limited by both inert structures and by the contractile portion of the muscle. Muscle reflexes are important when trying to stretch muscles, while an adequate warm-up is needed to make the tissues more pliable before we stretch. Following a warm-up, the body should be kept warm throughout the stretching period by using warm, loose-fitting clothing such as jog bottoms and a sweat shirt.

Five methods of flexibility training are generally used: *static, active, ballistic,* and two *PNF* methods.

Static stretching
Static stretching involves taking a limb to the point at which tightness is felt and holding this position. This is the sort of flexibility used in yoga, for example. As the position is held, the inert structures gradually elongate, while the muscle reflexes detect tension in the muscle tendon and gradually allow the muscle to relax. This is a particularly safe method of stretching, but because the position is held for up to 30 seconds the starting position chosen for the exercise must be comfortable and well supported. Lying and sitting on a mat are good starting positions, but kneeling and single leg standing are not. Once the position is achieved, concentration on breathing out and 'sighing' can allow the muscle to relax further. When the stretch is released, the muscle tension must come off slowly without allowing the tissues to 'spring' back.

Active stretching
Active stretching involves an active contraction (isometric or concentric) of one muscle to full inner range, requiring the antagonist to stretch fully to outer range. This is the type of stretching required in most sports for developing flexibility and strength at the same time. In addition, it requires good control so it enhances skill. This type of flexibility is most common in ballet and martial arts. An example is standing, holding on to a wall-bar for support, and actively flexing the hip slowly to its maximum range while keeping the knee locked.

Ballistic stretching
Ballistic stretching involves repeated small bounces at the end of the range of movement. Two factors are important here. First, when the whole body or trunk is used, the weight of the body moving at speed will build up momentum. The energy contained within the momentum can make it impossible to stop the movement soon enough, tissues are overstretched, and repeated small tears can occur called microtrauma. Over the years this can cause a build-up of scar tissue, altering the

mechanics of a joint. Second, the stretch reflex dictates that a rapid stretch will cause muscles to contract and tighten. Instead of increasing range of motion, the range may then actually reduce. It becomes obvious that this type of stretching is both dangerous and ineffective in most situations.

However, ballistic stretching can have an important role when carried out under the supervision of a physiotherapist after injury. The reason is that many sports, such as the martial arts, actually involve full-range actions and a high degree of flexibility. If the actions are performed slowly they are active flexibility actions, but when performed explosively – as they often are competitively – they become ballistic actions. The athlete practising this sport does not get injured each time he kicks simply because he has trained his body to re-set the stretch reflex so that it does not occur at the speed at which he is kicking.

If the athlete should suffer an injury, however, he must regain lost strength and flexibility and gradually reintroduce ballistic flexibility before he attempts competitive sport once more. This must be done in a highly controlled and supervised manner. Initially only mid-range movements are used, then gradually the range of motion is increased over many training sessions. It must be emphasised that full static, active and PNF flexibility, and full strength and power should be regained before any ballistic actions are used. The danger comes when inexperienced athletes try to copy a person who has been training with this type of action for many years. The body of the inexperienced athlete has not had time to adapt itself to these highly specialised actions so injury is the frequent outcome.

PNF stretching (1): contract–relax
PNF (proprioceptive neuromuscular facilitation) stretching is a method adapted from physiotherapy treatment of patients who have had strokes. It involves a series of movements designed to get the maximum out of a muscle by using primitive muscle reflexes. The first technique is called *contract–relax* (CR). With this method the athlete must first contract the muscle to be stretched and hold the contraction for 10–20 seconds. During this period the golgi tendon organs will register the tension build-up and cause autogenic inhibition, allowing an increased range of motion to be achieved. Because the muscle is tensed isometrically this technique is also called *post-isometric relaxation* (PIR).

PNF stretching (2): contract–relax–agonist–contract
The other method of PNF stretching is called contract–relax–agonist–contract (CRAC)). This consists of the contract–relax method first, but goes further by using the fact that when one muscle contracts, its opposing neighbour (the antagonist) must relax. This reflex, called *reciprocal innervation* (*see* page 26), allows us to stretch still further. To perform the CRAC method, the muscle to be stretched is first contracted and held for 20 seconds. This muscle is then relaxed, a brief pause is allowed, and then the opposing muscle is contracted to pull further into the stretched position. This has the added benefit of strengthening the muscle group that controls the range of motion, but can be difficult for some individuals to practise unsupervised.

All static and PNF stretching can be illustrated by a straight leg raise movement to stretch the hamstrings (*see* page 115). The individual lies on a mat and flexes the hip, keeping the knee locked. A training partner then presses the leg further into flexion and holds the new position to perform a static stretch. If the individual now presses the leg down on to the shoulder of their training partner, holds the hamstrings tight and then relaxes before the stretch is applied, he is applying CR. If, while the stretch is being applied, the individual pulls the straight leg into further flexion, trying to help their training partner, he is using CRAC.

Starting positions

The starting position for any stretching exercise is important both in terms of safety and effectiveness. It must allow free movement of the part of the body that is to be stretched, and it must be stable. An unstable position can cause an individual to lose balance and, therefore, lose control of a movement, placing excessive strain on the tissues being stretched. In addition, positions which are uncomfortable do not allow individuals to relax completely, and excessive tension in a muscle is not conducive to effective stretching. Furthermore, some individuals with medical conditions will find that certain starting positions, which place excessive or unbalanced stress on a weakened part of the body are unsuitable. Table 4.3 shows a variety of common starting positions with points to note and suggested modifications.

Partner work

Stretching can be done individually, but is sometimes more effective when performed with a partner. On the plus side, motivation is better; but on the minus side, the situation is less controlled because two people are involved. In each case a stable starting position must be chosen, with no chance of either person falling and violently increasing the stretch. The two partners act as one unit, so their combined mass has a single base of support and line of gravity (*see* pages 3–5). The base of support must therefore be larger than it would be for a single person. The person applying the stretch must move into a comfortable position that they can easily maintain,

rather than move into an awkward position that places them off balance or is uncomfortable, requiring them to continuously readjust their position.

The person who is being stretched must control the range of motion by giving continuous feedback. The techniques used must be fully explained to both partners, and they must both agree on the amount of pressure and length of hold that will be used. Initially, only minimal pressure should be used to increase the stretch. Pressure should not be exerted over a joint or an area of bone which may be painful – for example, the kneecap.

If partner activities are applied in a group exercise situation they must be practised under the supervision of an experienced and skilled instructor. Close supervision of individuals in the group is essential, especially when dealing with young or inexperienced individuals. When teaching partner work to adolescents, they should be matched for body-size and degree of flexibility.

Use of apparatus

Any form of training requires the body to be overloaded sufficiently to cause an adaptation. In the case of stretching exercises the overload is to increase the range of motion and hold the position. This is normally achieved manually, but apparatus may be used. Most commonly, a towel or belt is used to support the part of the body being stretched and to allow greater relaxation. For example, when a subject is quite inflexible, thigh stretches (*see* page 96) are sometimes easier if a towel is placed around the foot. Belts and pads may be used to keep the spine straight when hip exercises are used as there is a tendency to allow the spine to round, increasing lumbar stress.

Various machines are available to facilitate adductor stretches in the hope of achieving the

Table 4.3 Starting positions

Starting position	Points to note	Modifications
Standing	Individuals must stand in an erect and balanced posture. Common errors are to stand in a slumped or round-shouldered posture which does not allow correct spinal movement. With the feet together the position is unstable, especially if an individual has poor balance. The body-weight must be taken equally through both legs.	Standing with feet apart (stride standing), or with one foot in front of the other (walk standing), facing the direction of movement. Improve stability further by holding on to an object (support standing).
Walk standing (one foot in front of the other) Step standing (one foot up on a step)	Both positions are more stable than standing alone, but excessive stress may be placed on the knee if leg alignment is not correct. Ensure that the knee passes directly over the middle of the foot on the leading leg.	Use the thigh of the leading leg to lean on for support.
Supine lying	If the hip flexors are tight the pelvis may be tilted forwards, increasing the lumbar lordosis and placing pressure on the lumbar spine (*see* page 62). In individuals who have little body fat and prominent pelvic bones, pressure from a hard floor on body prominences can be painful. Some elderly subjects find lying makes breathing difficult for them, and some with arthritis of the neck joints find lying without a pillow causes dizziness and nausea.	Always lie on a padded mat. Use a rolled towel beneath the lower spine for support. Raise the neck on a small pillor or folded towel for elderly subjects. Bend the knees (crook lying) to relax the hip flexors and reduce pressure on the lumbar spine.
Prone lying	Individuals must turn the head to one side to be able to breath freely, and this can place excessive stress on the neck if the position is held. Pressure over prominent pelvic bones can be painful, and male subjects may find testicular compression occurs. Those with patellar pain find compression on a hard surface extremely painful.	Always use a well-padded mat, and encourage male subjects to press testicles away from compression from the public bone. Place a rolled towel below the forehead to enable the subject to breathe freely without compressing the nose. Bend the knees and place a rolled towel beneath the ankles.

Starting position	Points to note	Modifications
Sitting	When the hips are flexed further than 45°, tightness in the hip tissues begins to tilt the pelvis and flatten the spine. Eventually the spine may round, giving backpain after prolonged periods. Holding the head too far forwards places stress on the neck and shoulder muscles.	Encourage individuals to 'sit tall' and avoid slumping. Sit with knees apart to allow pelvis to tilt freely and maintain the lumbar lordosis.
Kneeling	Pressure on the front of the knee is very painful. Kneeling on all fours (prone kneeling) may place stress on the wrist. Kneeling on the knees only (high kneeling) places increased stress on the patella and can be unstable.	Use a well-padded mat. Ensure that the knees are shoulder-width apart to aid stability. Hold on to an object when using high kneeling.

classic 'splits' position. These are normally hydraulic or ratchet devices that force the legs further into abduction. From the point of view of safety, the amount of force used and its point of application are of paramount importance. Forcing the hips into an abducted position can place an excessive stress on the hip tissues. Applying this force below the knee can stress the medial ligament of the knee by imposing an inward (valgus) stress on these structures.

Continuous passive motion (CPM) machines have been used in a hospital setting for a number of years, and these are now being seen in the sporting context. The machines are electrically powered, and move the joints through a specified range for a set period. The amount of force available makes it essential that these machines are used only under the direct supervision of a physiotherapist.

♦ Developing agility ♦

We have seen that fitness is composed of a number of components. Of these, flexibility – the ability to obtain a range of motion about a joint – is only one. Agility by comparison is the ability to use and control this range of motion. For this reason, good agility requires a number of fitness components: flexibility, strength, muscle endurance, skill, and speed. Agility is thus fundamental to good sports performance.

Agility exercises involve controlled movements through a full range of motion, and may be used individually or in a circuit training format. Examples include movements from dance, ballet, aerobics and gymnastics, together with sport-specific actions requiring a high degree of agility.

◆ Summary ◆

- Warming up has been shown to lessen the number of irregular heart beats and reduce the blood pressure during exercise. It will also make tissue more pliable and affect psychological arousal.
- During a warm-up the movements to be practised during a workout should be rehearsed.
- Both active (exercise) and passive (heating) warm-ups may be used.
- When the body is exposed to a physical stress greater than the stress experienced in normal everyday activities, it is said to be overloaded.
- In 20 days total rest stamina reduces by 25% and strength by 35%.
- Training specificity means that the change which takes place in the body as a result of exercise will closely match the type of exercise used.
- Three body types exist: mesomorph (muscular), endomorph (fatter) and ectomorph (thinner). We are all a mixture of these three types.
- Stretching may be active, passive, or ballistic.

Chapter 5

Posture

♦ Why is posture ♦ important?

Posture is simply the relationship (alignment) between different parts of the body. Posture is important from two standpoints. First, good posture underlies all exercise techniques. Exercises started from a basis of poor posture tend to be awkward and clumsy with unequal tension placed on some body tissues. This can eventually lead to the accumulation of stress and consequent overuse injuries. Second, postural stress in daily life overworks some tissues and underworks others, leading to an imbalance of flexibility and strength. In the short term this imbalance gives rise to postural pain; but in the long term, because joints are pulled out of alignment, altered joint mechanics can lead to the development of joint surface degeneration (*see* fig 5.1).

Posture is maintained by both muscles and non-contractile tissues. A good posture is one in which the different parts of the body are correctly aligned, thus placing the minimum amount of stress on the body tissues. A good posture requires little muscle activity, so it is more relaxed and needs less energy to maintain it. At the same time, joint structures are not overstretched or shortened so much that they cause strain. In both of these cases a good posture is one that is balanced.

Two types of posture are important. Static posture is that seen at rest, while dynamic posture is that of motion – the type of body position a person takes up when moving. Static posture may be assessed by close inspection of the body, but the study of dynamic posture requires in-depth training, and often the use of advanced laboratory facilities.

A number of factors interact to create a person's static posture. Body type (*see* page 45) and genetic make-up are important, as are strength and flexibility. In addition, the way a person sees themselves (their body image) and the mental state of an individual will affect posture.

An individual cannot easily alter their bony make-up, so the posture with which they were genetically endowed is largely permanent unless surgically changed. Children, for example, who have particular spinal deformities often require a number of complex operations to straighten the spine. Similarly, bone or skeletal 'frame size' is constant for an individual, so a stretching programme must take this into account.

The important factor in the development of both flexibility and strength is *symmetry*. An unequal development of either of these two elements can pull the body out of alignment, causing postural faults.

The balance between postural muscles and movement muscles (*see* page 33) is also important. Postural muscles hold us up against gravity and include those trunk muscles which give us 'core stability'. Movement muscles will create great power and are able to move rapidly, but will tend to tighten. The combination of tightness (too much tone)

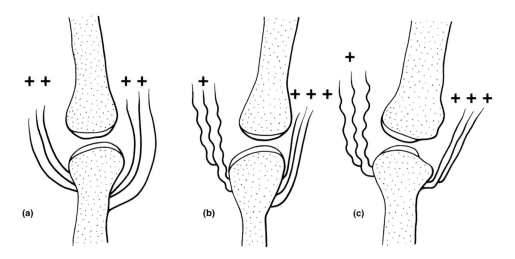

Figure 5.1 Muscle imbalance altering joint mechanics: (a) symmetrical muscle tone – normal joint; (b) unequal muscle pull (imbalance) – joint alignment poor; (c) joint surface degeneration

of some muscles and sagging (too little tone) of other muscles results in muscle imbalance which changes our postural alignment and gives rise to postural pain.

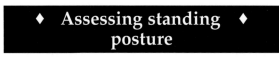

♦ Assessing standing ♦ posture

From behind

When the body is viewed from behind, with the feet three inches apart, a vertical line should divide it into two equal halves. The pelvic rims (anterior superior iliac spines) should be in the same horizontal plane, and the pubis and pelvic rims should be in the same vertical plane. An individual's posture can be assessed by comparison with a score-chart (*see* table 5.1). Anatomical 'landmarks' are compared with horizontal levels on the right and left sides of the body, and include: the knee creases, buttock creases, pelvic rim, angle of the shoulder blades, upper arm bones, ears, and skull protuberances. In addi-

tion, the alignment of the spinous processes and rib angles is observed. The distance between the arms and the trunk (keyhole), skin creases, and unequal muscle bulk are indicators of asymmetrical posture. Slight side bending of the spine (scoliosis) becomes more noticeable when an individual bends forwards (Adam's position) and a marked hump is seen over the twisted ribs.

Looking closely at the shoulder blade (scapula), the inner edge of the blade should be vertical and no more than three finger breadths from the spine. The blade should appear flat against the rib-cage, and no part of it should jut out or appear prominent. The appearance of the shoulder area on the right and left sides of the body should be roughly the same (symmetrical). The bulk of the muscles around the shoulder should be even, with no one area appearing either 'muscle bound' (excessive bulging) or 'wasted' (hollow). Finally, the contour of the muscle between the shoulder and neck (the upper fibres of the trapezius) should be smooth and rounded, rather than straight and tight like a cord.

Table 5.1 *Assessment of standing position from behind*

	Ear level – hair line
	Shoulder level – cervical spine
	Inferior angle of scapula
	Overall spinal alignment
	Keyhole
	Adam's position
	Skin creases
	Levels of pelvic rim, asis, belt line
	Buttock creases
	Knee creases Muscle bulk
	Mid-line Achilles angle
	Foot position

From the side

Standing posture is assessed by comparing it to a plumb-line or vertical line on a wall (*see* fig. 5.2). The line begins just in front of the outer ankle bone (lateral malleolus). In an ideal posture this line should pass just in front of the mid-line of the knee, and then through the hip, lumbar vertebrae, shoulder joint, cervical vertebrae, and the lobe of the ear. The chest is the furthest point forwards, and the buttocks are the furthest backwards. The posture is balanced and requires little muscle activity to maintain. When the body moves away from the plumb-line, stress is placed on the body tissues, and muscles have to work harder to maintain the unbalanced body position.

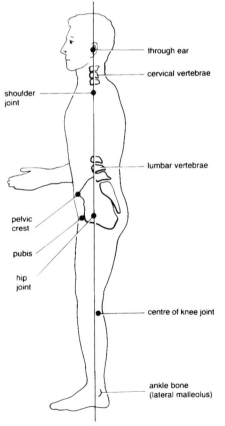

Figure 5.2 Posture plumb-line

Labels in figure: through ear; cervical vertebrae; shoulder joint; lumbar vertebrae; pelvic crest; pubis; hip joint; centre of knee joint; ankle bone (lateral malleolus)

The plumb-line posture assessment described above gives us an indication of segmental alignment. From this we can predict which muscles will have poor tone (sag) and which are likely to be tight and require stretching. More precise tests will enable us to be more accurate about which individual muscles are tight and therefore more objective with our exercise prescription.

Some of the most frequently used local clinical muscle tests are described below, and further tests are listed in Chapter 9. For all these tests, the client should be positioned ideally on an examination (massage) couch or gym bench. (For more detailed information on postural tests, *see* Norris, 1998.)

Thomas test

The Thomas test measures tightness in the hip flexors (iliopsoas and rectus femoris). The client lies on their back, with their knees bent and hanging over the end of the bench. From this position, both legs are fully flexed, bringing the knees to the chest and flattening the lumbar curve. The client holds one knee to their chest to maintain the lumbar position, and the other leg is lowered towards the horizontal, allowing the knee to extend (*see* fig. 5.3). The position of the femur and tibia indicates the muscle tightness.

If the femur rests above the horizontal, the hip flexors are tighter than is desirable. Either the iliopsoas or the rectus femoris could be affected, and straightening the knee will distinguish between the two. If straightening the leg allows the femur to drop down lower, the rectus is the tighter of the two muscles. This is because the rectus works over both the knee and the hip (the iliopsoas does not work

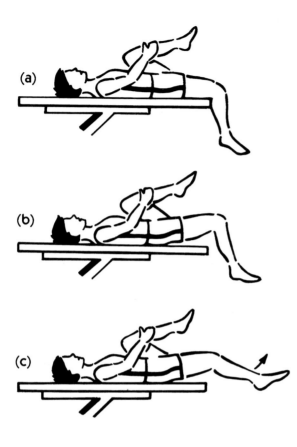

(a)

(b)

(c)

Figure 5.3 Thomas test: (a) knee is gripped to the chest and the opposite leg should touch the couch and show 90° flexion; (b) tight hip flexors; (c) tight abductors (ITB)

Ober test

The Ober test measures tightness in the hip abductors (ilio-tibial band and gluteals) and is named after Frank Ober who first described it in 1935. Essentially, the test aims to assess the length of the hip abductors while maintaining the neutral position of the pelvis in the frontal plane. The client lies on a bench on their side with the lower leg bent for comfort. The therapist stands behind them level with their pelvis (*see* fig. 5.4). The client's leg is abducted and extended to 15° and the pelvis is stabilised to prevent lateral tilting. The therapist presses down on the client's pelvic rim with their left hand angling the push towards the client's lower shoulder. The therapist's right hand supports the weight of the abducted upper leg. While preventing any pelvic movement, the upper leg is lowered down keeping it slightly back. Normally, the leg should lower to the horizontal position before any pelvic movement is detected. In an athlete, the leg should lower to the floor, indicating that the ITB and gluteals possess adequate flexibility. If the leg stops above the horizontal position, or if pelvic movement begins with the leg in this upper position, the ITB is tight. This test is also described in Chapter 8, exercise 53.

over the knee) and straightening the knee takes some of the stretch off the rectus. If the femur position remains unchanged, the iliopsoas is tighter than the rectus.

The knee, hip, and shoulder should also be in line. If the femur is abducted, the ilio-tibial band (ITB) is likely to be tight. Similarly the tibia should rest vertically. If it does not, tightness in the hip rotators may be indicated. This test is also described in Chapter 8, exercise 11.

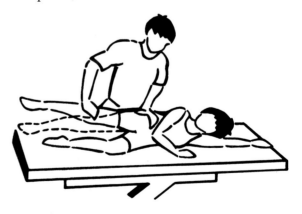

Figure 5.4 Ober test

Tripod test

There are many tests to assess the length of the hamstrings, including the straight leg raise and active knee extension exercises (*see* page 76). The tripod test, however, measures hamstring tightness, and the effect of any tightness on pelvic tilt and low back alignment.

The client sits on the edge of a bench with the feet unsupported. The spine is placed in its neutral position (*see* page 60) with the lower back slightly hollow. From this position one leg is straightened and the alignment of the lumbo-pelvic area is noted (*see* fig. 5.5). Ideally, the leg should be straightened to 70–80° while maintaining spinal alignment. Often, the leg cannot be fully straightened, and the spine sags into flexion, posteriorly tilting the pelvis and flexing the lumbar region. This is important because it indicates that tightness in the hamstrings is dictating spinal alignment and this is a common cause of postural back pain. As well as hamstring stretching exercises, core stability exercises should be practised to correct the fault (*see* pages 60–2).

Anterior chest test

Tightness in the pectorals and anterior deltoids will cause the shoulders to be pulled forwards and is assessed with the client lying on their back. Their arm is taken out to the side into a 'T' position (*see* fig. 5.6) and should rest ideally level with the bench. Taking the arm diagonally, so that it lies on the horizonal (frontal plane) and at 45° to the spine, will stress the sternal fibres of the pectoralis major and anterior deltoid (*see* fig. 5.6(b)). Taking the arm back to the 'T' position and then lowering the arm down the side of the bench, will stress the clavicular fibres of the pectoralis major (*see* fig. 5.6(c)). In this position, the arm should lie at 70–80° to the chest.

The shoulder can also be pulled forwards by tightness in the pectoralis minor, which attaches from the upper ribs to the corocoid process of the scapula. When this is the case, the back of the shoulder is pulled off the bench in supine lying. Normally the back of the shoulder should be no more than two to three finger breadths from the bench.

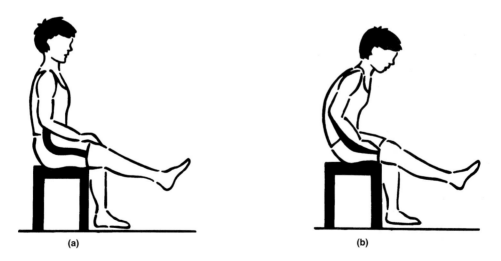

(a)   (b)

Figure 5.5 Tripod test: (a) pelvis level, leg straightens; (b) tight hamstrings cause backwards pelvic tilt and lumbar flexion

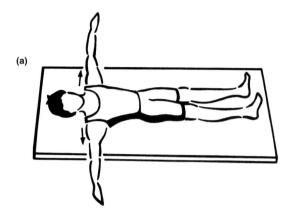

(a)

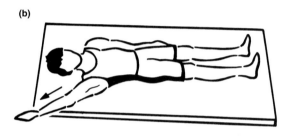

(b)

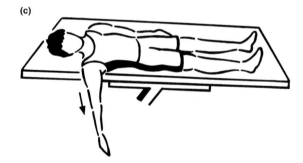

(c)

Figure 5.6 Anterior chest test: (a) 'T' position; (b) stressing the sternal fibres of pectoralis major and the anterior deltoid; (c) stressing the clavicular fibres of pectoralis major

Shoulder adductors

Tightness in the shoulder adductors (lattissimus dorsi and pectoralis major) will limit arm abduction. The latissimus is measured in a supine lying position. The arm is laterally rotated (because the muscle is a medial rotator) and abducted in an attempt to take it behind the ear. Normally the arm should rest flat on the couch (*see* fig. 5.7). Refer to the 'Anterior chest test' for assessment of the pectoralis major.

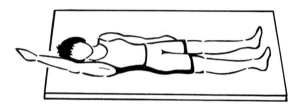

Figure 5.7 Measuring tightness in the latissimus dorsi: full abduction is combined with lateral rotation

♦ Postural faults and ♦ correction

Enhancing core stability

Before we begin to correct postural faults with stretching, we must ensure that an individual can hold firmly the origin of the muscles to be stretched. If this is not done, when we stretch, both ends of the muscle will move and alignment will be poor. Many of the large muscles of the lower limbs attach to the lumbo-pelvic region, while many muscles of the upper limbs attach to the scapula. Both of these areas must be stabilised before stretching begins.

The neutral spine position

The lumbo-pelvic region is stabilised by the deep abdominal muscles (transversus abdominis and internal oblique). Looking at figure 5.8, we can see that the superficial abdominals (rectus abdominis and external oblique) have fibres which run more or less vertically while the deep abdominals have largely horizonal fibres. When the muscles pull, therefore, the superficial abdominals will pull the pelvis to the rib-cage (flexion or rotation), while the deep abdominals will pull the abdominal wall to the spine and 'tighten the girdle'. In this way the deep abdominals are more able to stabilise the trunk and hold it in a 'neutral position' – mid-way between flexion (flat back)

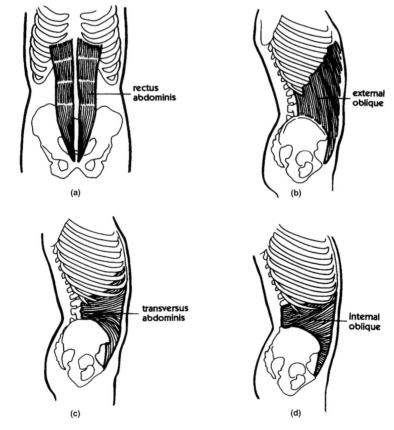

Figure 5.8 The abdominal muscles

and extension (hollow back) (*see* fig. 5.9). The neutral position aligns the lumbar tissues optimally and places least stress upon them.

When we move away from the neutral position, stress is increased. As we increase the hollow of the lumbar spine, the facet joints at the back of the spine are compressed. Over time, this can cause pain and joint damage, possibly leading to wear and tear of the joints themselves. If we reduce the hollow in the back, the spine is flexed and stress moves from the facet joints on to the disc. The flexion stress compresses the disc, tending to force it on to the nerves of the lower spine. This type of posture can give pain through nerve compression or nerve entrapment.

How to find your neutral spine position
To find the neutral position of the lower spine, we begin standing upright. Tilt the pelvis backwards, forcing your spine to flex (flatten) and then tilt your pelvis forwards, extending (hollowing) your spine. The neutral position

is mid-way between fully flattening and fully hollowing the spine. It should be the most comfortable position, depending on your posture type. (Posture types are discussed in detail later in this chapter.)

Core stability exercises

Having found the neutral position, we perform a series of simple exercises to re-educate the core stability muscles. First, we have to regain the hollowing function of the abdominals. Many people find this difficult initially, and tend to bend the spine instead.

Abdominal hollowing in standing
Start by standing with your back to a wall (*see* fig. 5.10). Focus your attention on your tummy button (umbilicus) and tighten your abdominal muscles to pull your tummy button in. A number of faults can occur when performing this exercise (*see* fig. 5.11). First, be

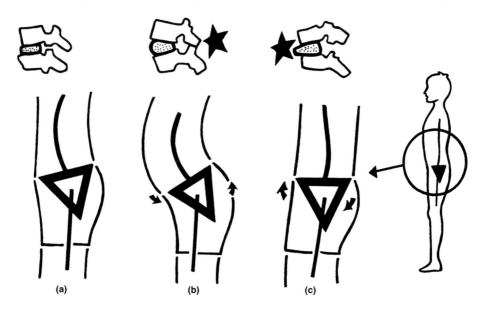

(a)   (b)   (c)

Figure 5.9 Neutral position of the lumbar spine: (a) neutral position; (b) hollow back – facet joints compact; (c) flat back – disc is stressed

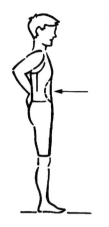

Figure 5.10 Abdominal hollowing in standing

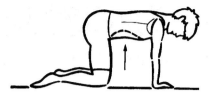

Figure 5.12 Abdominal hollowing in kneeling

Abdominal hollowing in kneeling

Allow your abdominal wall to sag down, and then pull it tight and up as if trying to touch your tummy button on to your spine. Again, make sure it is only your abdominal wall which is moving. Do not move your spine or hips (*see* fig. 5.12).

Heel slide

When you have mastered the abdominal hollowing exercises, you are ready to hold your spine stable against resistance. In the heel slide (*see* fig. 5.13), the hip flexor muscles are pulling on your spine, trying to move it away from the neutral position, while you are using your deep abdominal muscles to try to prevent the movement and maintain stability.

careful not to take a deep breath or hold your breath, and do not flex the spine. If you look at your lower ribs, they should not move throughout the hollowing action. If the ribs are drawn down, the superficial abdominals are working instead of the deep abdominals. If the ribs lift up, you are simply taking a deep breath and pulling your abdominal wall tight using respiration rather than abdominal muscle action.

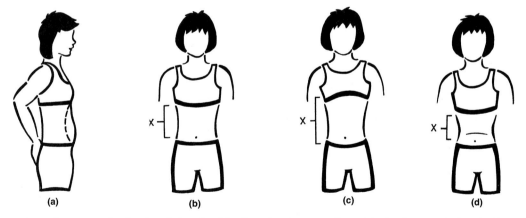

Figure 5.11 Common faults in abdominal hollowing in standing: (a) the lower abdominals only are pulled in, the ribs should not move; (b) the distance from the lower ribs to the pelvis (X) remains unchanged; (c) taking a deep breath: the ribs move up, increasing (X); (d) flexing the trunk, the ribs move down decreasing (X)

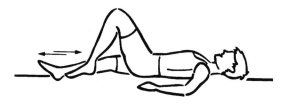

Figure 5.13 Heel slide

Lie down with your knees bent and place your finger tips over your lower abdomen. Pull your lower abdominals tight (hollowing) as before and keep them tight throughout the movement **without holding your breath**. Slide one of your legs out straight, making sure that your pelvis does not move and your spine does not hollow. You should aim to perform 10 slow repetitions on each leg, with each complete single leg movement taking about 10 seconds. No pelvic movement at all should occur throughout the whole exercise sequence.

To make it easier to spot unwanted pelvic movement, work with a partner. Place an adhesive marker on the front part of the upper lip of your pelvis (the anterior superior iliac spine) or mark it with a felt-tip pen. This will make it easier for your partner to detect even the smallest amount of pelvic movement.

Hollow-back posture

The lower part of the back (the lumbar spine) should normally be slightly hollow. This curve (the lumbar lordosis) is greatly affected by the tilt of the pelvis. The pelvis is balanced like a see-saw on the hip joints, and is controlled by the abdominal, spinal and hip muscles, and the ligaments that surround these areas. The abdominal muscles, working together with the gluteals and hamstrings, will tilt the pelvis backwards and flatten the lower spine, while the hip flexors and spinal extensors will tilt the pelvis forwards and increase the lumbar curve.

Pelvic crossed syndrome

In many cases an imbalance of these muscles exists, known as the *pelvic crossed syndrome* (PCS). Here we see a combination of excessive length and weakness in the abdominal muscles and gluteals (sagging) and tightness in the spinal extensors and iliopsoas (*see* fig. 5.14). The pelvis is seen to tip forwards, pulling the lumbar spine into an increased curvature or lordosis. This, in turn, causes stress to the small facet joints deep within the lumbar spine. This is the classic 'beer belly' posture, also seen after pregnancy and as a result of abdominal surgery.

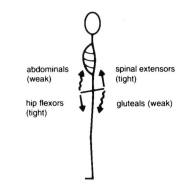

Figure 5.14 The pelvic crossed syndrome (PCS)

The weakness of the gluteal muscles has an important bearing on walking and running. Normally, as we take a step and the hip moves into extension, the gluteal muscles contract powerfully to push the body forwards. However, in PCS these muscles are weak and so are unable to propel the body correctly. To compensate for this, the hamstring muscles contract in an attempt to do the work of the gluteals (the hamstrings eventually becoming tight themselves). Because the hamstrings are not as strong as the gluteals, the action of hip extension is weaker. The body tries to make up for this by extending the lumbar spine instead of the hip, and again stress is placed on the lumbar region. The appearance now when running, stepping and walking is of a 'duck waddle' around the pelvic region.

How to correct the pelvic crossed syndrome

To correct this syndrome we cannot simply strengthen the gluteal muscles, because the imbalance affects all the hip muscles. Instead we must first focus our attention on stretching the tight hip flexor muscles. We saw on page 26 that there is a relationship between antagonistic pairs of muscles: when one muscle contracts, its opposite must relax. In the case of the hip muscles, the tight hip flexors have greater muscle tone and, therefore, may actually reduce the potential tone and strength of the hip extensors which lie opposite. This action of reducing tone by 'inhibition' (less nerve impulses reaching the muscle) is also known as *pseudoparesis* and is an important factor in balancing muscle pull around a joint. In the case of PCS we must stretch the iliopsoas and hamstrings (*see* table 5.2, (a) and (b)) while maintaining a neutral spine position. Once this has been achieved, both the gluteals and the lower abdominal muscles must be re-strengthened to correct the pelvic tilt. It is important to work the abdominals in their inner range to shorten, rather than simply strengthen, the muscles. Details of abdominal work of this type may be found in *Abdominal Training* (Christopher M. Norris, A & C Black, London, 1997).

Kyphotic posture

Upper crossed syndrome

An imbalance pattern also exists around the shoulder girdle, known as the *upper crossed syndrome* (UCS). Here the upper trapezius, levator scapulae and pectoral muscles are tight, while the deep neck flexors and the lower scapular stabilisors (serratus anterior and lower trapezius) are inhibited and weak. The abnormal posture seen here is one in which the head is held forwards (poking chin) and the normal curve in the neck is flattened out. The head posture places stress on the neck tissues and frequent headaches can result. The shoulders are rounded and the scapulae move further apart. In some cases the scapulae can be seen standing prominent under the skin (winging). Tightness in the trapezius and levator scapulae is commonly seen as a straightening of the neck/shoulder line, where the muscles stand out like tight cords (*see* fig. 5.15). This posture is frequently seen in those who spend many hours slumped over a desk and do little exercise in their spare time.

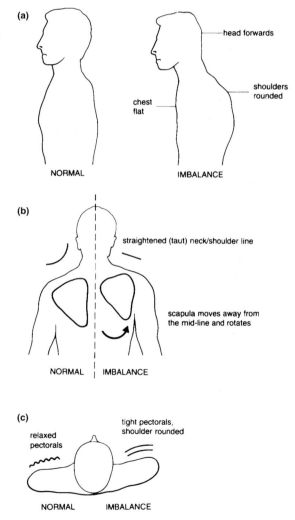

Figure 5.15 The upper crossed syndrome (UCS):

Table 5.2 Stretching exercises for posture

Problem		Exercise
(a) tight hip flexors		**iliopsoas:** hold on to an object for stability and press your hips forward
(b) tight hamstrings		**hamstrings:** hold behind one leg and straighten the leg
(c) head appears to be held forwards, poking chin		**chin tuck:** place hand on chin and gently slide head back horizontally
(d) tight band from neck to shoulder (upper trapezius), head appears tilted to one side		**side bend:** fix the shoulders by gripping a chair and pull the head in the opposite direction
(e) round shoulders		**'pec stretch':** stand in the corner of a room, place the arms on a wall and lean forwards
(f) flat low back		**low back:** push up on to the elbows
(g) tight back when bending forwards		**low back:** grip the knees into the chest

The altered muscular control of the scapulae causes them to twist slightly so that the shoulder socket (glenoid fossa) faces more vertically than normal. This means that the shoulder muscles must work harder to stop the joint from dislocating, and this additional work can give rise to a painful 'frozen shoulder' over time.

Although the shoulder girdle is a separate structure from the thoracic spine, the shoulder posture in UCS pulls the thoracic spine into excessive flexion, forcing the ribs together anteriorly and making breathing more difficult. In some cases, the thoracic vertebrae soften and develop incorrectly, a condition called Scheurmanns disease, which requires specialist treatment. In this case, the shoulder posture results from the spinal posture rather than the other way round.

How to correct upper crossed syndrome

Just as with the lower limbs, we begin the exercises by improving core stability. This time it is the stability of the shoulder blade (scapula) we are concerned with. It tends to ride up and outwards, and we need to pull it in the opposite direction. The first exercise (*see* fig. 5.16(a)) is to sit on a stool and ask your training partner to pull your shoulder into its optimal alignment. The shoulder blade is pulled down and in until its inner edge is vertical and the two blades are about 12–18 cm apart. You 'set' your shoulder muscles to hold this position as your training partner releases the shoulder blade. Try to hold the position for 10–30 seconds. For the next exercise (*see* fig. 5.16(b)), you try to correct your own posture and hold it. Again begin sitting, but try to lift your breastbone (sternum) without taking a deep breath. At the same time draw your shoulder blade in and down. Hold the position for 10–30 seconds as before, breathing normally.

When the kyphotic posture is created by tissue tightness alone, stretching is called for. Stretching is aimed at the neck (*see* table 5.2,

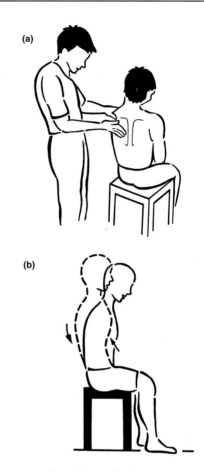

Figure 5.16 Shoulder stability exercises: (a) static repositioning; (b) sternal lift

(c)), the levator scapulae and upper trapezius (*see* table 5.2, (d)), and the pectoral and anterior deltoid muscles (*see* table 5.2, (e)). In each case, the scapula is stabilised in its optimal position (down and in) throughout the stretch.

In many cases the lordotic (hollow back) posture and the kyphotic posture may occur together (kypho-lordosis). This is because the increase in the lumbar lordosis results in an increased kyphosis to compensate which brings the body-weight back over the plumbline. If this is the case, exercise therapy must be aimed at both areas.

Sway-back posture

In a sway-back posture the whole pelvis moves forwards and the hips are forced into extension. While the pelvic tilt remains, the thoracic spine flexes and the lumbar lordosis is increased. This stresses the hip ligaments, and the ligaments on the front of the lower spine and behind the thoracic spine.

Comparing normal and sway-back postures (*see* fig. 5.17) we can see that in the case of normal posture the furthest point forwards is the chest, and the furthest backwards is the buttocks. In the case of sway-back posture the furthest point forwards is the abdomen and the furthest backwards is the thoracic spine. In the normal posture the lumbar curve is gently hollow along the whole length of the lumbar spine. In the sway-back, the hollow is sharp and more pronounced in the lower area. Finally, in the normal posture the spine

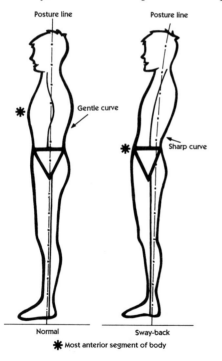

Figure 5.17 Sway-back posture

and legs are close to the plumb-line, but in the sway-back the spine and legs form a curve.

The sway-back tends to be a temporary 'slouching' posture, frequently seen in adolescents as they suddenly start to grow tall and 'shoot up'. However, it is still a cause of pain when held for longer periods. Correction involves tucking the chin in and lengthening the spine as though you were a puppet on a rope hanging from the ceiling. In addition, the chest should move forwards while the pelvis remains still. The easiest way to learn is by standing in front of a table and imagining the pelvis and chest as two toy building blocks sliding on top of each other (*see* fig. 5.18). The hips should not touch the table, and the chest should slide forwards as one unit, without altering spinal alignment.

Flat-back posture

The flat-back posture shows a markedly reduced lumbar lordosis, and is commonly seen following back pain when a person has rested in bed. The individual is unable to move the spine correctly, and most of the structures around it are stiff and sore. Stiffness may limit either flexion or extension, and the spine becomes almost fixed in a flat-back position. Stretching can help to alleviate the pain from this condition as the lost flexibility is gradually regained. The stretches should feel slightly uncomfortable, because they are working on very tight structures, however, they should not give back pain. If they do, exercise should be carried out only under the supervision of a physiotherapist.

With the flat-back posture the spine is gradually stretched into extension (*see* table 5.2, (f)). When forward bending is also limited, flexion stretches may be performed using the hips for leverage (*see* table 5.2, (g)). In each case, the movement is gently encouraged rather than being vigorously forced.

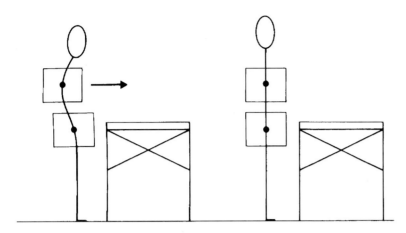

Figure 5.18 Correcting the sway-back posture

Postural faults in the lower limbs

Postural faults in the foot and leg can be detrimental to knee health, and stretching can help to alleviate the faults. We have seen that imbalance between the various hip and lumbar spine muscles can alter the way in which the hip is extended when walking and running. A further imbalance pattern also exists between the hip abductor and adductor muscles. The adductors show a tendency to tighten, and this in turn inhibits the hip abductors. The abductor muscles are important stabilisers of the pelvis as we lift one leg from the ground as in walking, stepping and running. As we lift the leg, the abductor muscles of the leg on the ground work hard to prevent the pelvis from dipping down. If these muscles are inhibited and weak, the pelvis dips causing a sideways 'duck waddle' (*see* fig. 5.19). This is most noticeable when performing step aerobics.

We saw in the PCS that when the hip extensors are weak the hamstring muscles work by substitution, and in so doing they become tight. In the case of weak hip abductors, the tensor fascia lata muscle works instead. This muscle attaches to the ilio-tibial band (ITB),

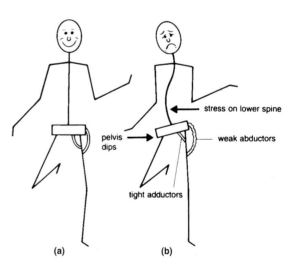

Figure 5.19 Weak hip abductors altering the stepping gait: (a) normal muscle balance – abductors and adductors are the same length and strength; (b) imbalance – tight hip adductors inhibit (weaken) abductors. As the opposite foot is lifted from the ground, weak abductors fail to support the pelvis, allowing it to dip down

which travels down the side of the leg. The ITB, in turn, has a connection to the side of the knee with a small slip to the kneecap itself. Because the tensor fascia lata is having to work too hard to cover up for the weakened hip abductors, it tightens the ITB and pulls the kneecap outwards as weight is taken on one leg. This is a very common cause of a painful kneecap, often seen in sport.

Correcting lower limb postural faults

The action now is clear. First, we must stretch the tight hip adductors. Then, if the condition has been present for some time, the ITB will be tight and will need to be stretched using the Ober test (*see* page 56). The test is performed, and the position of maximum stretch with the leg near the horizontal is held for 10–20 seconds. This should be practised daily with 5–8 repetitions.

To perfom this technique without a partner requires good lateral stability of the pelvis. This may be assessed using a 'hip hitching', or 'leg shortening', exercise (*see* fig. 5.20). In the side lying position the upper leg is again abducted and slightly extended. From this position the trunk side flexors are tightened by the hip hitching action. These muscles should remain tight, as the upper leg is lowered, to prevent any lateral tilting of the pelvis. The stretch is felt over the outside of the hip.

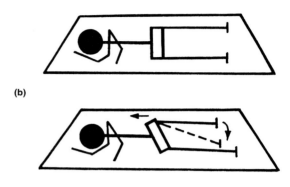

(b)

Figure 5.20 Self-stretch of tight hip abductors: (a) hip hitching in standing; (b) abductor stretch after hip hitching

♦ Summary ♦

- In a good posture the body segments are aligned to minimise joint stress.
- A good posture requires minimal muscle work to maintain.
- Posture is assessed with reference to a 'plumb-line' from behind and the side.
- Local tests of muscle tightness are used to determine postural problems in specific parts of the body.
- Posture correction begins by enhancing core stability.
- A muscle imbalance approach is used to stretch tight muscle and strengthen/ shorten lax muscle in order to realign body segments.

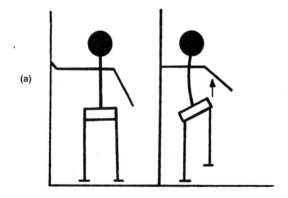

(a)

Chapter 6

Stretching the Nerves

Stretching exercises are generally said to affect the muscles with less affect on the joint tissues. However, an important structure which may be affected when performing stretching exercises is the nervous system.

An exercise which moves a limb will have effects on the nerves, as well as the muscles, and these effects must be considered when giving stretching exercises. As a limb is bent or straightened, the nerves must adapt. With elbow flexion, for example, the ulnar nerve is stretched while the radial and median nerves are shortened. In fact, from fully bending the elbow and wrist to fully straightening these structures, nerves may change their length by as much as 20%. Any stretching exercise we perform will have effects on nerves, and through them on other tissues seemingly unconnected to the body-part we are using.

♦ Structure of the nervous ♦ system

The nervous system can be visualised as an 'H' turned on its side, with the central bar of the 'H' being the spinal cord and the crossbars the nerves to the arms and legs. This structure is often divided into the central nervous system (CNS), consisting of the brain and spinal cord, and the peripheral nervous system, consisting of the nerves in the legs and arms. However, this division is misleading, because structurally many of the tissues within the nervous system are connected with each other, and the chemical reactions and electrical impulses within the nervous system travel its entire length. The nervous system can, therefore, be considered as a 'continuous tissue tract', a little like a single piece of string looping through the spine and limbs. Any tension (pulling) on one part will be transmitted throughout the whole structure and will have effects at points distant to the original site of disruption.

There are two types of nerve cells in nervous tissue: those which carry electrical nerve impulses (neurons), and those which protect and support the delicate conducting structures of the nervous system (neuroglial cells). In the limbs, the peripheral nervous system consists of neurons, which have a cell body and longs arms stretching out into the limb (*see* fig. 6.1). The cell body is located close to the spine, with the cell's arm stretching the whole length of the limb. For example, a single nerve cell may stretch from the lumbar spine along the whole length of the leg to the big toe! The cell's arm (axon) is covered with an insulating material called myelin which is produced from the neuroglial cells. The structure of the axon can be compared to an electrical cable of copper wire covered with insulating rubber. The nerve cells are grouped into bundles (fascicles) and the bundles are covered by a variety of membranes, the innermost being the endoneurium.

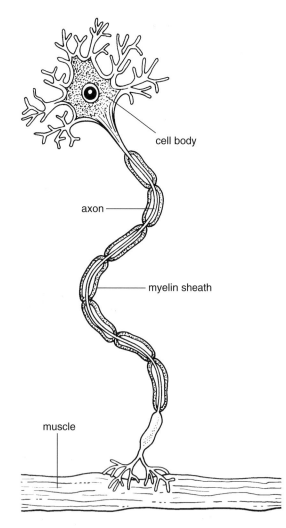

Figure 6.1 Structure of a nerve cell

In the central nervous system, the brain connects to the spinal cord at the base of the skull, and from the cord 'nerve roots' arise at 'T' junctions. Several nerve roots may come together to form a peripheral nerve travelling into the limbs. The cord, nerve root, and peripheral nerve each have a protective covering, but that of the nerve root is different to the other two structures. In addition, the point at which the nerve root leaves the spinal cord is very close to the vertibral bones themselves,

so the space is restricted. The combination of restricted space and poorer protection leaves the nerve root exposed to stress from certain movements and back injuries.

Attached alongside the spinal cord is the autonomic nervous system (part of the peripheral nervous system and consisting of sympathetic and parasympathetic parts), which provides the nervous control of the internal body environment, regulating, for example, heart rate and blood pressure. In addition, it controls aspects of the skin such as sweating and skin blood flow. Involvement of the autonomic nervous system in injury may, for example, cause whiteness in the skin with feelings of hot and cold, and sweating.

♦ Biomechanics of the ♦ nervous system

When nerves are stretched, they can do only one of two things: they can lengthen or 'give', or they can develop tension. Tension development is in the form of compression of the tissues and fluids contained in the nerve sheaths.

Movement of the nervous system may occur as a whole (gross movement), as in the case of a nerve sliding through a bony tunnel on the outside of the elbow. This movement may also be quite large: in the case of the spinal cord moving from full extension to full flexion, the cord can lengthen by nearly 10 cm, most of the movement being in the cervical and lumbar regions with little movement in the thoracic spine. With traction used by physiotherapists, a 5 kg stretching force can elongate the cervical spine by 10 mm and therefore stretch the spinal cord. Compression caused by carrying heavy weights will similarly compress the spine.

The nervous system, however, does not move consistently along its whole length as tension points occur (*see* fig. 6.2). These are at the level of the sixth cervical vertibra, the sixth thoracic vertibra, and the fourth lumbar vertibra. With flexion, *tethering* (attachment) at these points means the spinal cord will be stretched towards the neck and lumbar spine, but away from the thoracic spine.

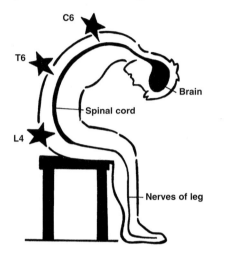

Figure 6.2 Tension points in the nervous sytem

Parts of the nervous system can also move in relation to others, a process known as *intra-neural movement*. For example, the spinal cord can slide within its containing sheath (dura mater), one nerve fibre within a bundle may move in relation to another, or an individual fibre may move in relation to its own sheath. In lateral flexion of the spine the convex side of the spinal cord stretches in relation to the other, the difference in length being as much as 15%.

In the case of gross movement, an injury which causes bruising or swelling over a region of the body may cause the nerve passing through this region to become adhered to other tissues. These types of injuries can range from bruising from a simple muscle pull affecting a nerve as its passes through the muscle, for example the sciatic nerve in rela-

tion to the hamstrings, to callus from a healing bone growing around the nerve, as in the case of the ulna nerve travelling around the outside of the elbow. These types of tethering will give nerve irritation and/or pain whenever the region is placed on stretch until the nerve breaks free. Intraneural movement may be limited if a crush injury causes swelling and scarring to regions of the nerve itself. If the individual nerve fibres within a bundle can no longer slide in relation to each other as a nerve is stretched around a corner, for example bending the knee, tension and pain may result.

◆ Vulnerable areas of the ◆ nervous system

Nerves have several vulnerable areas (*see* fig. 6.3).

Anatomical tunnels
There are tunnels formed through or around bone or soft tissues, which have relatively rigid walls and are therefore unyielding. Excessive movement may cause a build-up of friction, especially in the presence of swelling within the tunnel from a minor injury. An example of a nerve tunnel is the median nerve travelling through the tunnel made by the small wrist (carpel) bones. The area, called the *carpel tunnel* can give rise to 'carpel tunnel syndrome', a condition in which pressure on the medial nerve as it travels into the wrist gives aching and tingling sensations in the hand.

Nerve branches
A nerve is at risk when it branches, especially when this branching construction forms an acute angle. An example of this configuration is the digital nerve branching into the fourth and fifth toes. Pressure on this area through

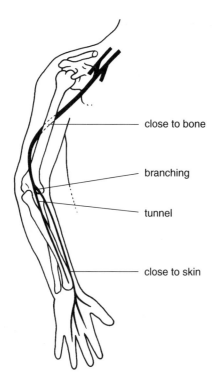

close to bone

branching

tunnel

close to skin

Figure 6.3 Vulnerable areas of a typical nerve

incorrect footwear can cause tissue tension and the development of a small cyst called a *digital neuroma*. This painful condition gives a burning sensation in the fourth and fifth toes due to nerve pressure.

Fixation points

The fixation points of the nervous system will not allow the normal sliding of nerves against underlying tissues and pressure near these points will be poorly tolerated. An example of a fixation point is at the head of the fibula bone where the common peroneal nerve wraps itself around it. Damage to this area is common, for example from a direct blow from a football boot or hockey ball. The resultant swelling and scarring tethers the nerve giving symptoms of injury.

Friction points

At certain points the nerves pass over or close to unyielding structures. Any tension will cause the nerve to give, but this will be limited. An example is where the brachial nerves extend from the cervical spine and pass over the first rib before travelling into the arm. Carrying heavy shopping bags can pull the nerves down on to the rib giving pain and tingling in the whole arm (brachial neuralgia).

Tension points

The classic tension points of the nervous system (*see* fig. 6.2) will cause the movement direction of the nerves to change, and are potential areas of concern. The sixth thoracic vertibra and the posterior aspect of the knee are examples, and these points are frequently a source of neural pain when stretching (*see* table 6.1).

◆ Effects of stretching the ◆ nervous system

Stretching a nerve has many effects: some that aid healing, and some that can be damaging.

Healing effects

After an injury that causes swelling, a nerve stretch will move the nerve past the swollen area preventing the clotted swelling from sticking (adhering) to the nerve. In addition, any swelling within the nerve between its individual fibres may also be dispersed by pressure changes brought about through rhythmic stretching. Following chronic injury, a nerve may become tethered to underlying structures: stretching may break the nerve free of its binding scar tissue and allow nerve impulses to pass unimpeded once more. Rhythmic movement will also improve the blood supply to the nerve, and with it the amount of oxygen reaching the nervous tissue. In addition, the transport system within the nerve, called *axonal transport*, will be improved by movement and reduced by prolonged inactivity.

Damaging effects

Repeated stretching

As with muscle and bone, the physical stresses involved with repeated stretching will cause minor injury (microtrauma) which will encourage the tissue to adapt and become stronger. However, caution is necessary with repeated microtrauma: if the degree of physical stress exceeds the capacity of the nerve (or any tissue) to adapt, tissue breakdown and injury may result.

Continuous stretching

When a nerve is stretched continuously, for example by poor posture, its blood flow may be impaired. As the stretch is placed on, the blood vessels supplying the nerve become thinner. With just 8% lengthening of the nerve, blood flow to the nerve begins to reduce substantially, and when the nerve is stretched by 15%, the blood flow is completely cut off. If this happens only once, or if the nerve is released, allowed to recover, and then stretched again, no problem will arise.

However, prolonged blood flow reduction can cause problems. Initially, the reduction in blood flow causes the blood within the vessels to stagnate, and all the oxygen within it is rapidly used up. This oxygen starvation is known as *hypoxia*, and the result is often pain and pins and needles which reduces when the blood flow is reinstated. Crossing the legs for prolonged periods in the cinema is a good example of neural hypoxia. When the legs are released, a shower of pins and needles ensues, followed by warmth and a return of normal sensation when full oxygen levels are rebuilt. If the hypoxia remains, however, permanent injury may result: the lining of the small blood capillaries is damaged and proteins

Anatomical tunnels	A tunnel has relatively rigid, unyielding walls and, therefore, the nerve is susceptable to pressure, e.g. median nerve travelling through the wrist (carpel tunnel).
Nerve branches	When a nerve branches at an acute angle its gliding mechanism is reduced. There is, therefore, less movement available to it, e.g. digital nerve branching into the fourth and fifth toes.
Fixation points	Fixation points are less yielding and nerves are more likely to be injured by tension at these points, e.g. common peroneal nerve wrapping around the head of the fibula.
Friction points	Where a nerve passes close to unyielding tissues, there is an increased likelihood of pressure, e.g. brachial plexus nerves passing over the first rib.
Tension points	Points where the direction of neural movement is reversed, e.g. sixth thoracic vertebra and posterior aspect of the knee.

Table 6.1 Vulnerable areas of the nervous system

leak out into the surrounding area, causing a change in fluid pressure leading to local swelling, which being unable to escape, spreads along the length of the nerve. The swelling may eventually clot causing a build-up of scar tissue within the area. The scarring will often stick to surrounding structures preventing the nerve from sliding properly with everyday movements, and causing friction as the nerve passes through tunnels and across other structures. More damage and nerve irritation occurs and pain is the inevitable result. In this way, minimal damage is exacerbated and a minor problem in one area spreads, causing symptoms in other body-parts.

Prolonged stretching

Stretching over a prolonged period may actually cause the nerve to lengthen. Hamstring stretching, for example, may cause the sciatic nerve to lengthen permanently.

◆ How to stretch the nerves ◆

A number of positions will cause tension build-up in the nervous tissue. Sometimes these positions are similar to classic stretches, and on other occasions they add subtle changes to a movement to apply a further stretch. In all cases, it must be remembered that nerves are delicate structures that must be treated with respect. Any nerve stretch may cause not just a feeling of tightness and aching, but pins and needles as well. This indicates that a stretch is working, but is too harsh. If this occurs, the stretch should be released slightly so that the feeling is just short of producing pins and needles. Over time, as the nerve stretches further, the point at which pins and needles occurs will move further away as the range of motion possible is increased.

Most of the stretches detailed below are combinations of several movements. When a nerve is adhered and causing problems, the stretch should begin with the distal movement, away from the tight structures. For example, if a combination of trunk flexion, straightening the leg and pulling the foot up (*see* the slump exercise below) causes problems in someone who is recovering from low back pain, the stretch should be released by allowing the knee to bend and the back to straighten slightly. Further stretch is gradually added by firstly pulling the foot up into dorsiflexion, and then straightening the knee. Only at the last moment should the hip be flexed or the trunk bent further. After stretching, nervous tissue will need to recover in the same way that a muscle does. Remember that stretching a nerve reduces its blood flow, so adequate recovery must be allowed for. For this reason, nerve stretches should only be practised on alternate days, and a gentle warmth and general feeling of stretch is all that is required. Nerve stretches which cause pain are too extreme.

Slump

This action stretches the whole of the nervous system, affecting the spinal cord, upper limb nerves and lower limb nerves.

Starting position and instructions (A)

Sit on a stool and link your arms behind your back. Gently flex your spine beginning with your neck. At the same time straighten one of your legs, moving your foot up and your leg into a horizontal position (*see* fig. 6.4).

Starting position and instructions (B)

Sit on the edge of a table with your feet together and unsupported. Link your hands behind you, and gently flex your spine beginning with your neck, taking your chin down

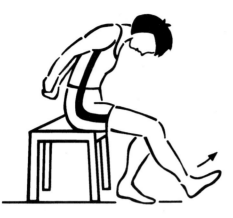

Figure 6.4 Slump

to your chest. Continue the movement, rolling through the spine rather than leaning forwards. At the same time, straighten both legs, locking the knees and pulling the feet towards you. Maintain the full stretch for 30 seconds and then slowly release.

Variations
Components of this action may be used individually and built-up into a full sequence. If one leg is very tight, keep that knee bent and gradually work towards straightening it, easing into the tightness but not forcing the movement. This may be achieved by placing the tight leg on top of the other and using the lower leg to provide a passive stretch while the upper leg relaxes. Alternatively support the foot of the tight leg on the floor by placing it on a shiny piece of paper. With the weight of the leg taken through the floor, slide the foot forwards and backwards, again gradually working towards the fully extended position.

Long sitting slump

A long sitting slump increases the emphasis on the thoracic spine.

Starting position and instructions
The exercise is best performed close to a wall, with the feet pressed against the wall to dorsiflex them. Keeping the legs locked out straight, place your hands beside your knees and gradually flex the spine, beginning with the chin to the chest and rolling through the spine aiming the head towards the hips rather than the knees (*see* fig. 6.5).

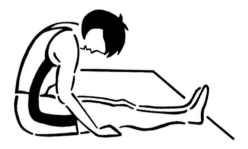

Figure 6.5 Long sitting slump

Variations
The rollover, or plough, places greater pressure on the thoracic spine and further forces the stretch (*see* fig. 6.6). This is a specialised neural stretch that is contraindicated in a general exercise programme. If you have a history of lower back pain, you should only attempt it after consulting a physiotherapist. Lie on the floor on your back and bring your legs up over your head leaving your arms on the floor. Pull your feet towards you (dorsiflexion) and straighten your legs. Try to place your toes on the floor to take some of your body-weight or use one or two cushions to rest the feet on.

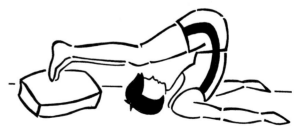

Figure 6.6 Rollover (plough)

Straight leg raising

The straight leg raising (SLR) movement is used as a test when a person has back pain. The aim is to see if the action produces pain from the back into the buttock and down the leg into the foot. If this is the case, it follows that the sciatic nerve is trapped and this is caused frequently by an intervertibral disc that has bulged or burst into the path of the nerve root at its junction with the spinal cord. The SLR action is a good illustration of the various stages of nerve movement that occur as a stretching exercise is performed (*see* fig. 6.7).

Starting position and instructions
Lie on the floor and flex one hip, slowly raising the leg. As the leg is raised initially, the sciatic nerve slides through a notch in the pelvis; as the leg is raised further, between 20–30° of hip flexion, the nerve roots start to move past the individual vertebrae. Movement of the nerve past neighbouring structures stops altogether as the leg is raised past 70°. From this position to the full range stretch of 90°, the nerve is stretched like an elastic band.

Sliding of the nerve, therefore, occurs below 70° with stretching only coming on from this range to the end of the straight leg raise movement. The SLR action is useful to mobilise and then stretch the sciatic nerve when its normal free motion is reduced, frequently as a result of previous back pain.

Variations
A modification of the SLR action that is also used to stretch the sciatic nerve is active knee extension (*see* fig. 6.8). This is a popular hamstring stretch, but with minor adjustments it will also place considerable stress on the sciatic nerve passing down the leg. Lie on the floor on your back, flex one of your hips and knees and place your hands behind your knee. Straighten the leg, keeping the knee directly above the hip. Greater stress is placed on the nerve, rather than the hamstring muscles, by medially rotating the hip and pulling the foot towards the body (dorsiflexion).

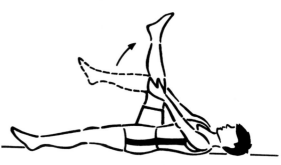

Figure 6.8 Active knee extension

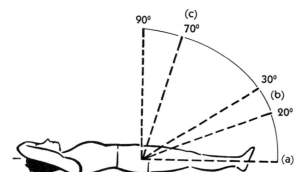

Figure 6.7 Effects of straight leg raising (SLR): (a) movement of sciatic nerve begins at the pelvis; (b) movement of roots begins at the spine; (c) minimal movement only, but increase in tension

Another alternative is to use a doorway (*see* fig. 6.9). The heel slides up the wall, the weight of the leg being partially supported, and again the foot is dorsiflexed. Overpressure from the hand on to the knee is useful to encourage the last few degrees of movement. The full stretch should be held for 30 seconds. As a progression, both legs may be stretched at once by placing them on a wall.

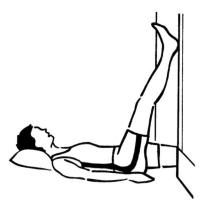

Figure 6.9 The straight leg raising (SLR) in an open doorway

Quadriceps

The femoral nerve of the leg may be stretched with the quadriceps muscles (*see* fig. 6.10).

Starting position and instructions
Standing, flex one of your knees and pull the hip back into extension. Normally, the trunk is kept upright to emphasise the effect on the quadriceps, but to increase the involvement of the femoral nerve, flex the trunk and bring the chin down to the chest. This stretch is a variation of the rectus femoris stretch described in Chapter 8, exercise 5.

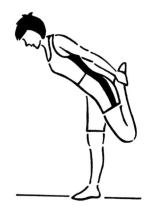

Figure 6.10 Variation of quadriceps stretch for the femoral nerve

Upper limb tension

In the arm, three nerves need to be stretched: the radial nerve, medial nerve, and ulnar nerve. Since all three come from the spinal cord in the thoracic region, they form a meshwork of nerve roots called the brachial plexus. The nerves of the brachial plexus can be stretched by the upper limb tension test (ULTT) in the same way as the SLR stretches the lower limb nerves. In addition, several variations can be used to throw stress on to single nerves when this is required. The ULTT combines shoulder depression with abduction to 90°. The elbow is then extended and the wrist extended later. The head is rotated and side flexed away from the stretched arm. This action is normally carried out passively on a patient by a physiotherapist, but may also be performed as a stretch.

Starting position and instructions
Standing side on to a wall, place your hand on the wall at shoulder height, and slowly turn the body and head away from the wall (*see* fig. 6.11). Pressing down on the stretched shoulder (depression) with the other hand will increase the stretch further.

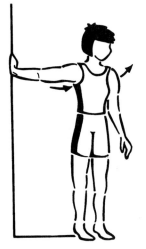

Figure 6.11 Upper limb tension test (ULLT)

Variations

The radial and medial nerves may be stretched with the arm by the side of the body. The shoulder girdle is depressed, the arm turned outwards (laterally rotated at the shoulder and supinated at the forearm) and wrist extended to stretch the medial nerve. To stretch the radial nerve, the arm is inwardly rotated and pronated while the wrist is flexed (*see* fig. 6.12).

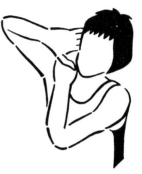

Figure 6.13 Ulnar nerve stretch of the right arm

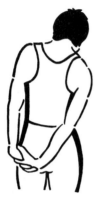

Figure 6.12 Radial nerve stretch of the left arm

The ulnar nerve is individually stretched by depressing the shoulder girdle, abducting the arm and flexing the elbow. The wrist is then extended, as though placing the flat of the hand over the ear (*see* fig. 6.13). If the ulnar nerve is very tight, pins and needles will be felt on the outside of the elbow over the 'funny bone'.

♦ Summary ♦

- There are two types of nerve cell: those that carry electrical impulses and those that protect and support the nerves.
- All the nerves and the spinal cord are linked into a 'continuous tissue tract'.
- Nerves will slide as a limb is stretched.
- After injury sticky swelling will 'tether' a nerve reducing its normal movement.
- A nerve has several vulnerable areas where it may be trapped or its movement restricted.
- When a nerve is stretched, its blood flow is reduced. Repeated nerve stretches should therefore be avoided.
- Nerve stretching exercises resemble muscle stretches, but with subtle changes. They must be exact.

Chapter 7

Stretching Research

In this chapter we will look at some of the research which has been conducted on aspects of stretching covered in the rest of the book. Research is ongoing, so knowledge in this subject area is ever increasing. Full details of recent research papers are listed in 'References' on pages 152–3, for readers seeking further information. New material is also available from the 'Update' sheet on the Norris Associates web site: http://www. norris @ndirect. co.uk.

◆ Stretching and posture ◆

1 In a lordotic posture, the pelvis is anteriorly tilted and 'hangs on the hamstrings' (*see* page 62). In this posture, the hamstrings are likely to be tight (increased tone), whereas in other postures their length is likely to be unrelated to pelvic tilt. Li et al. (1996) measured the importance of the length of the hamstrings. They took subjects with tight hamstrings who had a straight leg raise (SLR) of less than 70°, and then applied a stretching programme. They found that the SLR improved and the motion of the pelvis in forward bending changed. Interestingly, the static postural alignment of the pelvis did not alter. *Result*: the length of the hamstrings may well be more important to pelvic control during forward bending than to static posture.

2 The importance of the pelvic tilt position when performing a hamstring stretch was addressed by Sullivan et al. (1992). They took 20 subjects with tight hamstrings and used static stretching and PNF techniques in either anterior or posterior pelvic tilt. Each subject performed 10 minutes of stretching for four days per week over a two-week period. They found that the group who used a starting position of anterior pelvic tilt gained significantly greater hamstring flexibility. *Result*: anterior pelvic tilt was better for stretching regardless of the type of stretching used.

◆ Stretching and muscle ◆ stiffness

1 Halbertsma et al. (1996) looked at the load–deformation curve (*see* page 7) of stretched muscle. They took subjects with slightly short hamstrings (SLR less than 80°) and applied 10 minutes of static stretching for a single period. They found that the stress strain curves before and after exercise did not change, indicating that the stiffness of the muscle did not change in a single exercise bout, however, the range of motion increased. *Result*: stretch tolerance was improved by static stretching.

2 To measure the effect of stretching on muscle stiffness, McNair and Stanley (1996) used oscillation of the calf muscles. In their

experimental setup, subjects were seated, with a weight on the knee and their foot on a rocker mechanism which allowed the heel to drop down into dorsiflexion, prestretching the calf muscles. Another weight was then dropped on the knee to rapidly stretch the muscle further. An accelerometer was connected to the weight holder resting on the leg to measure vertical movement and oscillation. The small movements which occurred were amplified 100 times, and an EMG recording demonstrated that no voluntary muscle contraction was occurring. They found, firstly, that the elastic stiffness of the calf muscles reduced significantly after 10 minutes jogging at 60% of maximal heart rate; and that, secondly, the same effect was achieved after static stretching for 5 repetitions – holding each stretch for 30 seconds with a 30-second rest between each stretch. *Result*: a marked reduction in muscle stiffness can be brought about by static stretching.

3 Measuring the effect of tendon tap on the calf muscles was used to demonstrate the effect of stretching on muscle reflexes by Rosenbaum and Henning (1995). They showed improved muscle compliance after 3 minutes of static stretching of the calf muscles, and improved muscle force development and decreased EMG activity after a 10-minute warm-up run on a treadmill. *Result*: stretching produced muscle changes which would tend to reduce the risk of injury, while warm-up produced changes which would tend to enhance performance.

4 Magnusson et al. (1996) used the movement of an isokinetic dynamometer (passive torque) to measure the resistance of the hamstring muscles to stretch during passive knee extension. Passive torque is the force which a muscle exerts to 'push back' against the pressure of the machine. The subjects in the study stretched their hamstrings for 90

seconds 5 times, with a 30-second stretch between each repetition. During the static stretch, passive torque reduced indicating that the muscles were 'giving' a little. The stiffness of the muscles was also shown to reduce, but both measures returned to normal within one hour of testing. *Result*: stretching was effective, but the timing of stretching in a workout and the need to stretch regularly is important.

◆ Stretching as part of ◆ a warm-up

A warm-up will result in a number of physiological factors which may be of benefit to stretching:

1 Elevated temperature improves a person's ability to perform physical work in general. The critical level at which various metabolic chemical reactions occur is lower so the reactions occur sooner (Bergh and Ekblom 1979).

2 Muscle contraction is more rapid and more forceful (Bergh 1980). The sensitivity of nerve receptors and the speed at which a nerve is able to transmit its impulse is quicker (Astrand and Rodahl 1986). The improvements in nerve conduction seen after a warm-up are particularly important for PNF stretching, for example, where reflex mechanisms are used to improve range of motion.

3 The stiffness (viscosity) of the synovial fluid limits a joint's range and ease of motion. The viscosity of the synovial fluid is reduced (it offers less resistance) as its temperature rises during a warm-up (Astrand and Rodahl 1986). A greater force and length of stretch is required to tear muscle which has undergone a warm-up due to the reduction in viscosity of the connective tissue within the muscle

(Safran et al. 1988). LaBan (1962) showed a 1.5% increase in the length of a stretched tendon following a temperature increase to 42.5°C while later, Warren et al. (1971) demonstrated that tendon heated to 45°C increased in length by 5.8% and its force to failure was 58% greater than that at a normal body temperature. Realistically, these extreme temperatures, compared to body temperature of 38.9°C, can only be achieved through passive heating as used by a physiotherapist. However, they do demonstrate the importance of allowing tissue to warm before it is stretched.

♦ Injury prevention and ♦ performance enhancement

Many athletes believe that warm-up and stretching will help to prevent injury and make them perform better. If stretching can offer less resistance to movement and increase range of motion, it is possible to see that a mechanism may exist to justify these claims. However, because there are many factors which are interrelated with injury and performance, these claims are as yet to be substantiated.

1 The combination of warm-up and stretching has been shown by some authors to actually reduce the incidence of injury. Ekstrand et al. (1983) showed that a group of footballers performing a 20-minute warm-up, which included 10 minutes stretching, suffered only 75% of the injuries that their colleagues did. Stretching as part of a rehabilitation programme has been also been shown to reduce the rate of injury re-occurrence to only 1% following calf muscle injury (Millar 1976).

2 Stretching may improve the efficiency of movement in certain circumstances. In one study (Godges et al. 1989) the economy of running gait was shown to improve at both moderate and high exercise intensities through increases in hip range of motion. Other studies, however, have shown the reverse. Gleim et al. (1990) showed that 'tighter' subjects were significantly more economical as fast walkers and joggers than more flexible subjects. The tighter subjects also demonstrated better oxygen consumption values on treadmill activities.

♦ Muscle reflexes and ♦ stretching

The effects of stretching on reflexes is often investigated by measuring the excitability of a muscle. To do this, a *Hoffmann reflex* (H reflex) is used. We saw that when a muscle is stretched rapidly it responds by evoking a stretch reflex (*see* page 24). The Hoffman reflex is similar, except that it is an artificial reflex. If a muscle, usually the soleus in the calf, is electrically stimulated with a single shock, a muscle twitch results and is seen on an EMG machine. The strength of this muscle twitch (H reflex) is recorded as the height of the EMG signal graph. If a group of motor nerve cells (motor neuron pool) is more active (excitable) the H reflex will be stronger because more motor nerves are involved in the contraction.

A number of factors will influence the excitability of the motor neuron pool. For example, if a subject clenches their teeth by biting hard, the H reflex is stronger, demonstrating that the motor nerves to all muscle will be excited. Although there is no logical connection from the jaw to the calf, there is a functional relationship which is important to stretching. When we grip any muscle tightly, in this case the jaw, neural signals are sent not just to the muscle concerned, but along the spinal cord as well. This has the effect of 'setting' the muscles and bracing our posture to create stability. The effect, known as the *Jendrassik manoeuvre*, is important, because if we are trying to stretch a muscle using PNF techniques we want that muscle to relax and offer less resistance to the stretching force. If we place a subject in a starting position where they are unbalanced and gripping on to something, or where they feel insecure, the increased tone which results will have a knock-on effect to the tone of the muscle we are stretching, even though that muscle may be some distance away.

1 Research into the response of muscle to PNF stretching has used the H reflex to assess muscle excitability after isometric contraction using the contract–relax method (*see* page 47). Moore and Kukulka (1991) showed the H reflex to be suppressed after isometric contraction. The excitability of the motor nerve and the stretch reflex mechanism itself appears to decrease following isometric contractions, and this decreased level lasts for about 10 seconds, whether or not the muscle was contracted for 1 second or 30 seconds. This gives a 10-second 'window' in which to apply the stretch.

2 Looking at the EMG trace to judge the efficiency of the stretch reflex, Nicol et al. (1996) used a maximum vertical depth jump. They found that both reflex activity and muscle biochemistry changed considerably: creatine kinase activity increased showing micro-damage to the muscle fibres (as occurs with eccentric exercise); the stretch reflex sensitivity was reduced completely by the second day after exhaustive exercise; and recovery was not fully complete until four days after the exercise. *Result*: exhaustive exercise, especially that which is likely to cause muscle damage such as eccentric actions, reduces the sensitivity of the stretch reflex and may remove some of its protective function making injury more likely.

♦ Types of stretching ♦

Several researchers have asked the question, 'Which is the best way to stretch?' Static stretching seems to be as effective as ballistic stretching, except that ballistic stretching creates a considerable amount of muscle soreness (Etnyre and Abraham 1986). PNF techniques provide greater improvements in range of motion than either static or ballistic methods (Enoka 1994).

Webright et al. (1997) compared static stretching with active stretching. They took 40 subjects through a stretching programme in the sitting position. Initially, subjects were unable to lock their knee (minimum of $15°$ short of full extension) when sitting with the femur at $90°$ and statically stretching the hamstrings. One group practised static stretching (single repetition held for 30 seconds) while the other practiced slow (non-ballistic) active knee extension (30 repetitions each taking 1 second). Each group performed two bouts of stretching daily for six weeks. The result showed that both groups developed an equal amount of flexibility with subjects changing from $15°$ short of full extension to $8–10°$ short of full extension. Importantly, this programme demonstrated significant increases in flexibility through a short (30 second) stretching programme performed daily, in just six weeks.

♦ Stretches – how long and how many? ♦

The exact amount of time needed to effectively stretch has been the subject of many studies.

1 Bandy and Irion (1994) used knee extension to test static stretch timing. They chose 47 subjects with limited knee extension and subjected them to 15-, 30-, or 60-second static stretches. Each group stretched for five days a week for six weeks. Their results showed that both the 30- and 60-second stretches were more effective than the 15-second stretch, but importantly the 60-second stretch gave no greater gains than the 30-second one. The conclusion they made was that there is no advantage in holding a stretch for 60 seconds, 30 seconds seems to be an adequate period to hold a static stretch.

2 Because the effects of stretching are cumulative (*see* page 42), a number of repetitions are normally performed. Taylor et al. (1990) found that the greatest effects of stretch to the muscle and tendon occurred during the first four stretches with greater number of repetitions failing to produce greater improvements. In this case, more did not seem to be better!

◆ Limiting factors in range ◆ of movement

1 Two factors will limit the possible range of motion available at a joint: contractile and non-contractile structures (*see* pages 43–4). The degree of limitation presented by the various tissues varies between joints. In the spine, Adams et al. (1980) looked at cadavers and found that the vertebral disc limits flexion and extension movements by 29%, while the supraspinous and interspinous ligaments limit the same movement by 19%. The facet joint capsules have the greatest limitation to movement, at 39% For the metacarpophalangeal joints, the capsule limits movement by 47%, muscle by 41%, tendons by 10%, and skin by 2% (Johns and Wright 1992).

2 When muscles are relaxed, the improvement in range of motion with each successive stretch will increase. Taylor et al. (1990) used the extensor digitorum longus muscle in the leg, stretched it by a set amount and held the stretch for 30 seconds. Each bout of stretches consisted of 10 repetitions. Two outcomes emerged from this research: firstly, to produce the same resistance force, the muscle had to be stretched further by 3.5%; and, secondly, when the muscle was stretched to a pre-set length, the load required to do this gradually reduced. The conclusion is that over time, the passive resistance offered by muscle to a stretch reduces. Thus static or PNF stretching seems to be more effective than ballistic. In addition, each stretch should be *held* and the individual stretches *repeated* for a set of 10 or more repetitions.

◆ Summary ◆

- The angle of pelvic tilt is important for the application of stretches around the hip, especially for the hamstrings.
- Stretching reduces the 'stiffness' in a muscle in much the same way as a warm-up.
- Muscle reflexes are important to the stretching process.
- A 30-second static stretch is most effective, and four or five repetitions only should be applied.

Table 8.1(b) Trunk

Joint movement	Muscles stretched
Extension	Rectus abdominis, external oblique, internal oblique, psoas minor, psoas major
Rotation	Multifidus, rotatores, semispinalis, internal oblique, external oblique
Lateral flexion	Quadratus lumborum, intertransversarii, external oblique, internal oblique, rectus abdominis, erector spinae, multifidus
Flexion	Quadratus lumborum, multifidus, semispinalis, erector spinae, interspinales

Table 8.1(c) Lower limb

Joint movement	Muscles stretched
Hip flexion	Gluteus maximus, hamstrings (semitendinosus, semimembranosus, biceps femoris)
Hip adduction	Gluteus maximus, gluteus medius, gluteus minimus, tensor fascia lata
Hip abduction	Adductor magnus, adductor longus, adductor brevis, gracilis, pectineus
Hip extension	Psoas major, iliacus, rectus femoris, sartorius, pectineus
Hip lateral (outward) rotation	Anterior part of gluteus medius, anterior part of gluteus minimus, tensor fascia lata, psoas major, iliacus
Hip medial (inward) rotation	Gluteus maximus, piriformis, obturator internus, gemellus superior, gemellus inferior, quadratus femoris, obturator externus

Knee joint extension	Hamstrings (semitendinosus, semimembranosus, biceps femoris), gastrocnemius, gracilis, sartorius
Knee joint flexion	Quadriceps femoris (rectus femoris, vastus lateralis, vastus intermedius, vastus medialis), tensor fascia lata

Ankle joint dorsiflexion	Gastrocnemius, soleus, plantaris, peroneus longus, tibialis posterior, flexor digitorum longus, flexor hallucis longus
Ankle joint plantarflexion	Tibialis anterior, extensor digitorum longus, extensor hallucis longus, peroneus tertius

◆ Beginner ◆

Exercise 1 • Hip adductors — long sitting

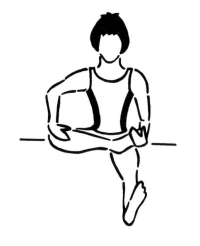

Starting position and instructions

Sit on the floor with both legs straight. Flex your right leg, placing your foot on your left thigh above the knee. Support the foot with your left hand, and press down on the knee with your right hand. Lengthen your spine and maintain spinal alignment throughout the movement.

Variations

Start by sitting with your back flat against a wall and a rolled towel placed in the small of your back (lumbar area) to maintain spinal alignment. You can also sit on a wedge to anteriorly tilt the pelvis.

Coaching points

Most individuals are asymmetrical and will find one leg is more flexible than the other. There is a tendency with this exercise for those who have reduced flexibility of the adductors, to tilt the body towards the bent knee lifting the pelvis and buttock (ischial) from the floor. This gives an apparent increase in flexibility as the knee is able to be lowered further, but there is no greater stretch placed on the adductors.

Exercise 2 • Gluteals

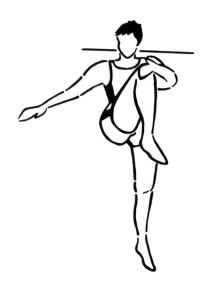

Starting position and instructions

Lie on the floor with the left leg straight. Flex the right knee and pull it upwards and across towards the left shoulder.

Variations

Pulling the knee across the body rather than towards the shoulder will vary the emphasis of the stretch.

Coaching points

This exercise also places stress on the pelvis so it is inappropriate after pregnancy.

Exercise 3 • Hamstrings – long sitting

Exercise 4 • Hamstrings (active knee extension)

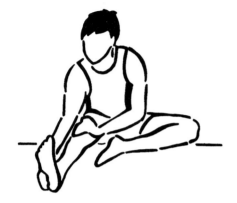

Starting position and instructions

Sit with your right leg straight and your left leg comfortably bent. Reach forwards with the right hand to grip the sole of your right foot. Press your left hand on your right knee to maintain knee extension. Maintain spinal alignment, gently curving throughout the whole spine.

Variations

Place both hands on the right knee, lengthen your spine and hinge only from the hip avoiding spinal flexion.

Coaching points

Individuals who are hyperflexible in the thoracic spine may place excessive stress on this area. To avoid this, retract the shoulders, expand the chest and maintain this position throughout the exercise.

Starting position and instructions

Lie on the floor with the left leg straight and flex the right knee and hip to 90°. Grip your hands behind the right knee and actively straighten the leg using your quadriceps muscles. The knee should remain directly above the hip.

Variations

Place your hand on the front of the leg and actively push your leg on to your hand using the power of your hip flexors; at the same time extend your knee. This will cause the hamstring muscles to further relax through reflex action.

Coaching points

Pulling the toes towards you and flexing your neck will throw stress on to the neural tissues and sciatic nerve and away from the hamstrings (*see* page 76).

Exercise 5 · Rectus femoris – standing

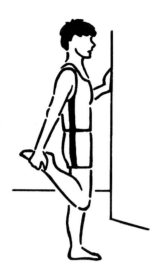

Starting position and instructions
Stand side-on to a wall with your left hand supporting your body-weight. Flex your right leg, and grip your ankle with your knee flexed. Pull your right hip back into extension, while maintaining correct spinal alignment.

Variations
Loop a towel around your ankle to reduce the amount of knee flexion and to allow you to pull into further hip extension, which will emphasise the upper portion of the muscle.

Coaching points
This exercise also stretches the femoral nerve (*see* page 77).

Exercise 6 · Calves (a)

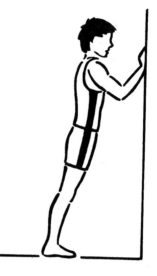

Starting position and instructions
Begin facing a wall with both feet together, arms straight and hands on the wall. Keeping your legs straight, bend your arms to lower your trunk towards the wall.

Variations
Walking towards and away from the wall will change the emphasis of the exercise.

Coaching points
Asymmetry is common in this area so you may find that one arm can bend more than the other.

Exercise 7 · Calves (b)

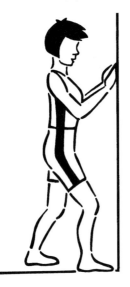

Starting position and instructions
Begin facing a wall in a half lunge position with your right foot forward. Place your hands on the wall and bend your arms to lower your body-weight forwards, pressing your right foot into dorsiflexion.

Variations
Altering the angle of the foot away from the perpendicular will change the emphasis on the gastrocnemius muscle.

Coaching points
The heel must remain on the floor throughout the movement.

Exercise 8 · Lower back flexion

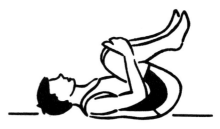

Starting position and instructions
Lie on the floor, drawing your knees up to your chest. Grip your knees and pull them into your chest and up towards your shoulders, creating a rocking position in your lower spine. This movement stretches the erector spinae.

Variations
This movement may be combined with rotation or lateral flexion to alter the stress on your spine.

Coaching points
The movement is one of pulling your knees towards your shoulders rather than pulling your knees in towards your chest alone.

Exercise 9 · Thoracic spine – kneeling

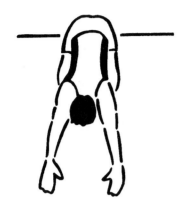

Starting position and instructions
Kneeling on all fours, sit back on your ankles, keeping your hands fixed. Feel the stretch in the latissimus dorsi and thoracolumbar fascia muscles and the thoracic spine.

Variations
Placing one knee slightly forwards of the other will impart some lateral flexion on your spine.

Coaching points
This position may be held for 30–120 seconds to gain full benefit of the stretch on your spine.

Exercise 10 · Shoulder rotation

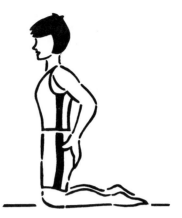

Starting position and instructions
Kneel and internally rotate and extend the shoulders to place your hands behind you on the small of your back. Draw your elbows back and together to stretch the external rotators and flexors of the shoulder (teres minor, supraspinatus, infraspinatus, deltoid and long head of the biceps muscles).

Variations
Moving the hands up towards the shoulders, or down towards the knees, will vary the site of stretch.

Coaching points
Optimal spinal alignment must be maintained through this exercise. The lumbar spine must not be hyperextended.

♦ Intermediate ♦

Exercise 11 · Hip flexors (Thomas test)

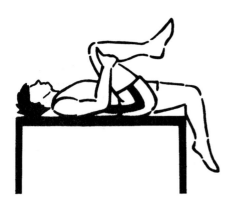

Starting position and instructions
Lie on a bench with the left leg over the bench end. Flex the right hip and knee and pull the knee towards the chest.

Variations
Begin with both knees bent and the feet flat on the bench. Pull one knee to the chest and then lower the opposite leg.

Coaching points
This is a basic clinical test of hip flexor tightness in the iliopsoas and rectus femoris of the lower leg: increasing the flexion at the knee emphasises the rectus femoris; reducing the knee flexion (straightening the leg) emphasises the iliopsoas.

Exercise 12 · Hip flexors (half lunge)

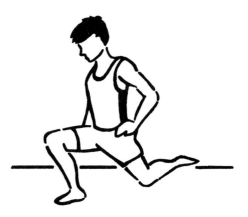

Starting position and instructions
Begin half kneeling with your right leg in front, and tighten your abdominal muscles to stabilise your trunk. Press your right leg forwards, forcing your left hip into extension.

Variations
Support your weight with one hand on a stool.

Coaching points
Altering the degree of hip rotation will change the emphasis on the hip flexors. Relaxing the abdominal muscles and allowing the pelvis to tilt anteriorly will give the impression of a greater range of motion at the hip, but, in fact, it will stress the lumbar spine.

Exercise 13 • Hip adductors — sitting (bilateral)

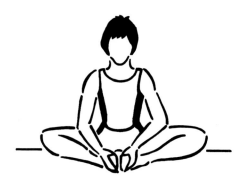

Starting position and instructions
Sit on the floor and place the soles of your feet together. Grip your feet and press down on your knees or thighs using your elbows. Maintain spinal alignment and try to lengthen your spine, reaching your head towards the ceiling as you press down with your elbows. Do not allow your pelvis to tilt backwards.

Variations
Sit on a wedge so that your pelvis is anteriorly tilted and your spine maintains its lumbar lordosis.

Coaching points
Because the adductor muscles are attached to the pubic bone there is a tendency with this exercise to posteriorly tilt the pelvis and bring the pubic bone forwards releasing the stretch from the muscle. When this is done the knee will lower further but there is no greater stretch placed on the adductors. Maintaining the lumbar lordosis and the neutral pelvic position is therefore essential.

Exercise 14 • Hip adductors (wide splits)

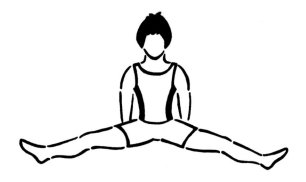

Starting position and instructions
Sit on the floor. Abduct your hips and place your hands on the floor behind your trunk. Press down with the hands to push the hips forwards, anteriorly tilting your pelvis to increase the stretch.

Variations
Sit with your back flat on the wall and flex and extend your feet to work your ankles further apart.

Coaching points
Make sure the ankles do not slide forwards, releasing the adductor stretch.

Exercise 15 · Hip adductors and lateral flexion

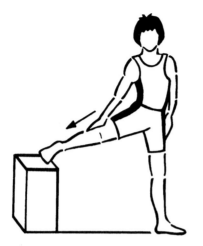

Starting position and instructions
Place your right foot on a waist-high object with your toes pointing forwards and laterally flex your trunk towards the right side.

Variations
Altering the height of the object will vary the stretch.

Coaching points
The exercise is unstable, because you are standing on one leg, so if you need to, hold on to an object throughout the movement. The upper arm must reach towards the foot, not press downwards on the outside of the knee. Because of the stress placed on the knee, this exercise is unsuitable if you have had a knee ligament injury.

Exercise 16 · Hamstrings and spine (sit and reach)

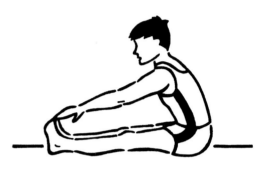

Starting position and instructions
Sit on the floor with your legs straight. Reach forwards to touch your toes, curling evenly through the whole of your spine. This exercise stretches the hamstrings and the spine. If an individual is hyperflexible in the thoracic spine, this area will take an excessive stretch. Spinal alignment must be maintained throughout the exercise.

Variations
Begin the exercise in the same position with a straight spine, press the chest forwards and retract the shoulders. Move only from the hips using a hinge action.

Coaching points
This modification reduces the forwards distance you reach, but increases the stretch on the hamstrings.

Exercise 17 • Hamstrings – sitting (using a stool)

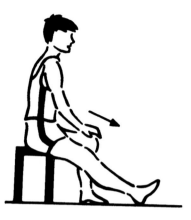

Starting position and instructions
Sit on a bench or stool that allows you to reach the floor with the right leg straight and the left leg bent. Anteriorly tilt your pelvis and keeping your spine straight reach forwards towards your knees. Support your body-weight through your arms throughout the exercise.

Variations
Pulling the foot and toes up towards you, and flexing the neck and spine will increase emphasis on the neural tissues and sciatic nerve.

Coaching points
Those who have had back pain may have tightness in the neural tissues or sciatic nerve which may cause pins and needles during this movement.

Exercise 18 • Hamstrings (using a stool)

Starting position and instructions
Stand in front of a waist-high stool and place your right foot on it. Keeping your right leg straight, lean forwards, moving from the hip while maintaining correct spinal alignment.

Variations
Hold on to an object or place your hand on a wall to increase the stability of the movement.

Coaching points
Pulling your toes towards you and flexing your head and trunk will increase the stretch on the neural tissues and take the stretch away from the hamstring muscles.

Exercise 19 · Hamstrings (using a bench)

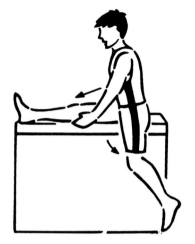

Exercise 20 · Rectus femoris – lying

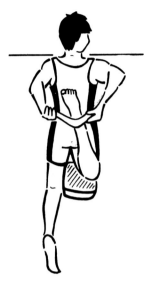

Starting position and instructions
Sit with the right leg straight along a bench, and the left leg flexed at the knee and pressed back into extension of the hip. Lean forwards, attempting to reach the foot of your right leg.

Variations
Releasing the full knee extension will increase the emphasis on the upper portion of the hamstrings.

Coaching points
The pelvis should not tilt when extending the hip; no more than 15° extension is required.

Starting position and instructions
Lie on the floor on your front and bend your right knee. Loop a towel around the right ankle and pull your knee into flexion, drawing your heel towards your buttock.

Variations
Place your knee on a block forcing the hip into extension. This emphasises the upper portion of the muscle.

Coaching points
The upper and lower portion of the muscle must be stretched equally.

Exercise 21 · Anterior tibials

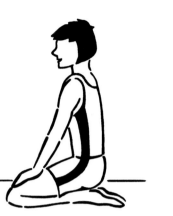

Starting position and instructions
Kneel, and then sit back on your ankles, pressing the anterior aspect of the ankle to the floor.

Variations
Place a folded towel beneath your toes to press them into flexion and increase the stretch on the toe extensors.

Coaching points
This exercise places considerable stress on the knees. Individuals with knee pain should perform the exercise beside a stool and take their body-weight through their hands on to the stool.

Exercise 22 · Lower back extension

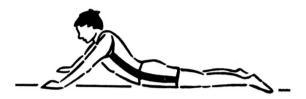

Starting position and instructions
Lie on the floor on your front, placing your hands on the floor in the 'press-up' position. Push with your arms to arch your spine, keeping your hips firmly on the floor. Pause in the upper position and then lower. This movement stretches the rectus abdominis muscle and corrects any pressure imbalance in the lower back discs from prolonged sitting or lifting.

Variations
Pushing from your forearms until your elbows are locked at 90° will limit the range of motion; pulling your arms towards your shoulders will increase the range of motion.

Coaching points
This movement should be encouraged rather than forced, and repeated rhythmically to gain a pumping action on the discs of your lower spine. You should feel the stretch, but not pain, in the lower back. If you experience pain, stop immediately.

Exercise 23 · Thoracic spine

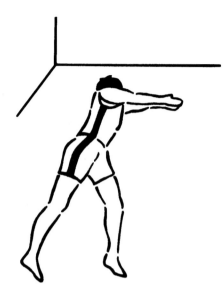

Starting position and instructions

Lie on the floor with your feet comfortably astride, and your arms out in a 'T' position. Stretch your right arm across your body and rotate your trunk to the right at the same time. This movement stretches the thoracic spine and the oblique abdominals and latissimus dorsi muscles of the upper side of the body.

Variations

Increasing the amount of abduction of your legs will increase the stability of the movement.

Coaching points

Keeping your hips still will increase the emphasis of the stretch on your thoracic spine.

Exercise 24 · Full spine rotation

Starting position and instructions

Stand with your feet astride and arms out in a 'T' position. Rotate to the right, leading with your right arm and then reverse the movement. This exercise stretches the oblique abdominals.

Variations

Lowering your arms and leading just with the shoulders reduces the overload.

Coaching points

The leverage and momentum from your arms make it essential that the movement is performed in a slow and controlled fashion.

Exercise 25 · Spinal rotation (using a stick)

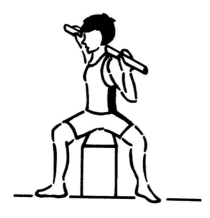

Starting position and instructions
Sit astride a bench with a stick across your shoulders. Grip the ends of the stick, and twist your trunk to the right, pressing your right elbow back and your left elbow forwards. This movement stretches the oblique abdominals.

Variations
Reaching your hands above your head before the stretch is commenced will pull harder on the thoracolumbar fascia.

Coaching points
This exercise must be performed slowly, with a hold at the end to avoid building up potentially damaging momentum.

Exercise 26 · Spinal rotation

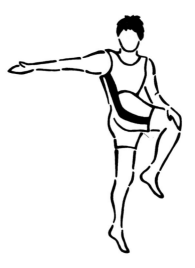

Starting position and instructions
Lie on the floor with your right arm out in a 'T' position. Flex your right knee and rotate the trunk towards the left leg, bringing your knee towards the floor. Place overpressure on the stretch by pressing your knee to the floor using your left arm. The main emphasis of this stretch is on the oblique abdominals, but it also stretches the latissimus dorsi and anterior deltoid of the horizontal arm.

Variations
Place a cushion on the floor and take your knee down on to the cushion. Altering the degree of flexion at your hip and knee will alter the stress of the stretch.

Coaching points
Because this action involves leverage it should be performed in a slow and controlled manner.

Exercise 27 · Spinal rotation (two legs)

Exercise 28 · Spinal rotation (assisted)

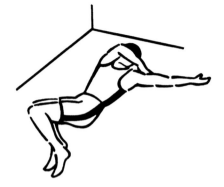

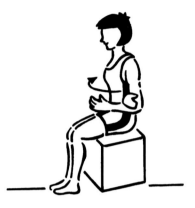

Starting position and instructions
Lie on the floor with your knees and hips flexed. Take your knees to the right side of your body and your arms to the left, maintaining the stretch. The main emphasis of this stretch is on the oblique abdominals, but it also stretches the latissimus dorsi and anterior deltoid of the upper arm.

Variations
Place a small cushion on the floor and lower your knees on to the cushion to reduce the range of motion.

Coaching points
Due to the weight of your legs, they should be lowered slowly. Dropping your legs is potentially dangerous to your spine.

Starting position and instructions
Sit on a low bench, place your right arm behind the small of your back and grip the elbow of your left arm. Twist to the right, leading the movement with the left hand. This exercise stretches the oblique abdominals.

Variations
If the subject is unable to hook the hand through the arm, a looped towel may be used around the elbow instead.

Coaching points
It is usual to have some degree of asymmetry so rotation to the right and left sides may not be equal.

Exercise 29 • Lateral flexion – standing

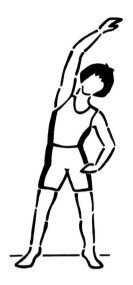

Exercise 30 • Lateral flexion (using a stick)

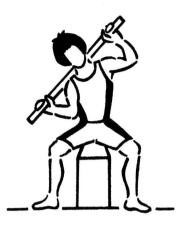

Starting position and instructions
Stand with your feet astride. Laterally flex your spine, placing your left arm on your waist, or thigh, to support your body-weight. Take your right arm above your head to increase the stretch. This movement stretches the latissimus dorsi and external oblique on the right side of the body.

Variations
Use both arms on the waist to reduce the overload.

Coaching points
Asymmetry of the lateral flexion of the spine is common so movements may not be equal on both sides.

Starting position and instructions
Sit astride a bench with a stick across your shoulders. Grip the ends of the stick, and laterally flex to the right, moving the stick upwards towards the ceiling. This movement stretches the external oblique and quadratus lumborum on the left side of the body.

Variations
A towel may be used instead of the stick if the shoulder is not flexible enough to allow the stick to be placed behind the neck.

Coaching points
Pure lateral flexion should be used rather than combining it with flexion or rotation.

Exercise 31 • Lateral flexion (with overpressure)

Exercise 32 • Trunk lateral shift

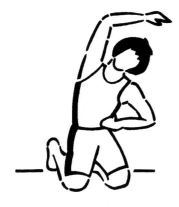

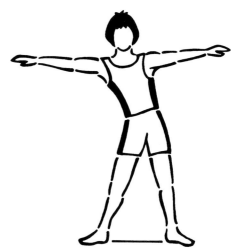

Starting position and instructions
Kneel on the floor and reach above your head with your right arm to lead a lateral flexion movement. Your left arm acts as a pivot by pressing the side of your rib-cage. This exercise stretches the external oblique and the quadratus lumborum on the right side of the body.

Variations
Instead of taking your arm above your head, place both arms on the hips to reduce the overload.

Coaching points
Asymmetry in this area is common so movements may not be equal on both sides.

Starting position and instructions
Stand with your arms out in a 'T' position. Lunge laterally with your right hand to shift the trunk. This exercise stretches the external oblique and quadratus lumborum on the left side of the body.

Variations
Performing the exercise with your back to the wall will ensure maximum alignment; performing in front of a mirror will often make it easier to control.

Coaching points
The movement should come from your hips with your shoulders remaining fairly static.

Exercise 33 · Rhomboids and thoracic spine

Exercise 34 · Anterior chest and shoulders

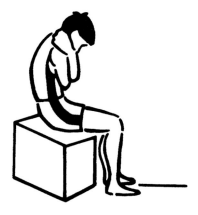

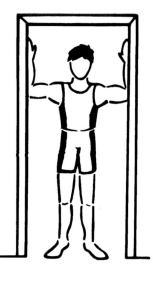

Starting position and instructions
Sitting on a bench, grip both arms across your chest, placing your hands on your shoulders, and flex the trunk at the thoracic spine.

Variations
Combine the flexion movement with rotation and/or lateral flexion to change the emphasis on the thoracic spine.

Coaching points
This exercise should be used with caution as this area is quite often too flexible (hyperflexible).

Starting position and instructions
Stand in front of a doorway in a room with your shoulders and elbows flexed to 90°. Lean forwards, pressing your chest through the doorway and forcing your arms back into extension.

Variations
Increasing and reducing the height of the arms will vary the site of stretch.

Coaching points
Because the full body-weight is being supported, heavy individuals, or those with poor shoulder flexibility, should take up a lunge position, moving some of the body-weight on to the front foot.

Exercise 35 · Upper trapezius

Exercise 36 · Shoulder adductors and extensors

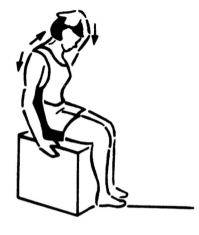

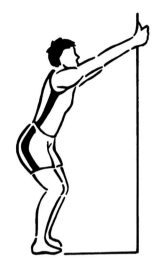

Starting position and instructions

Sit on a bench and grip the bench top with your right hand. Laterally flex your neck to the left allowing your right shoulder to elevate. Fix your neck in position with your left hand and actively depress your right shoulder to overload the stretch.

Variations

Flex and extend the head to change the emphasis of the stretch.

Coaching points

The power from the stretch must be from pulling the shoulder downwards rather than pulling on the neck, since the neck is the more delicate structure.

Starting position and instructions

Grip a high point and straighten your arms. Keeping your hands fixed, bend your knees and lower your body down and back, feeling the stretch beneath your arm. This movement stretches the latissimus dorsi and triceps muscles.

Variations

Altering the position of the hands will change the exact point of stretch

Coaching points

Gripping a higher point will increase the range of motion, but reduce the body-weight placed on the stretch. A lower point encourages the subject to lean back and take more weight through the shoulders.

Exercise 37 · Shoulder rotation – lying

Exercise 38 · Shoulder rotation (weight overload)

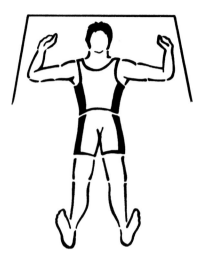

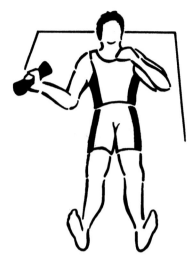

Starting position and instructions
Lie on the floor with your arms abducted and elbows flexed to 90°. Allow your forearms to fall back into the horizontal position, rotating the shoulders. This position stretches the shoulder rotators.

Variations
Alter the angle of abduction at the shoulder to vary the exact site of stretch.

Coaching points
With the use of weights, this exercise is ideal for contract–relax techniques.

Starting position and instructions
Lie on the floor and grip a weight bag in your right hand. Place your upper arm close to your body and flex your elbow to 90°. Allow the weight of the bag to force your shoulder into external rotation. This position stretches the shoulder rotators.

Variations
Increasing and reducing the weight will change the intensity of the stretch.

Coaching points
Since a weight is used, this exercise is ideal for contract–relax techniques.

Exercise 39 · Forearm pronation and wrist flexion

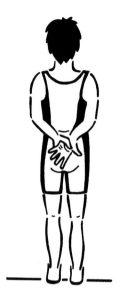

Starting position and instructions
Stand with your arms by your sides. Pronate your right forearm and flex your right wrist. Grip your right wrist with your left hand and press your right wrist into further flexion.

Variations
The exercise may be combined with radial or ulnar deviation to maximally stress your extensor carpi radialis longus muscle.

Coaching points
For cases of tennis elbow, combining the wrist flexion and ulnar deviation will maximally stress your extensor carpi radialis longus muscle.

Exercise 40 · Forearm pronation and supination (using a stick)

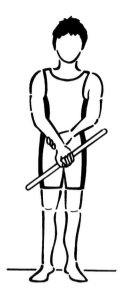

Starting position and instructions
Flex your right elbow and supinate your forearm. Gripping a stick in your hand, support your forearm in your cupped left hand. Pronate and supinate your right forearm, using the weight of the stick as overpressure.

Variations
Using a lighter or heavier stick will change the intensity of the stretch.

Coaching points
At the end of the range of motion holding the stretch will increase the overload.

Exercise 41 · Wrist extensors (a)

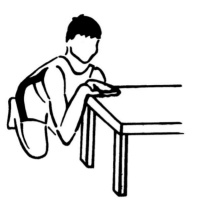

Starting position and instructions
Place your right hand at the edge of a low table and place your left hand on top of your right so your thumb is level with your wrist crease. Press the right forearm down into the vertical position, pressing your right wrist into extension. Use the weight from your left hand to keep the heel of your right hand on the table.

Variations
Altering the height of the table will vary the range of motion.

Coaching points
Where a single intercarpel joint is stiff, the movement may be localised by pressing the thumb of the left hand into the wrist crease of the right hand.

Exercise 42 · Wrist extensors (b)

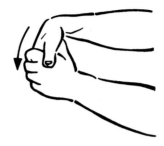

Starting position and instructions
Straighten your right arm and flex your right wrist. Grip your right hand with your left, placing your left thumb into your flexor wrist crease. Using your left thumb as a pivot, pull your right wrist into full flexion.

Variations
Altering the position of the thumb will localise the stretch.

Coaching points
Because of the leverage involved, the stretch must be slow and controlled.

Exercise 43 · Wrist extensors (c)

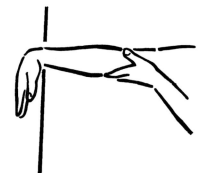

Starting position and instructions
Stand facing a wall, place the back of your right hand flat on the wall with your fingers vertical and straighten your arm. Use your left hand to lock your right elbow and maintain the locked position throughout the movement. Lean forwards towards the wall, pressing your wrist into further flexion.

Variations
Placing your hand higher up the wall will increase the range of motion.

Coaching points
Where an ache is felt close to the elbow, the muscle is being stretched, but where the sensation is over the wrist, the wrist extensor tendons and tissue are being stretched.

Exercise 44 · Wrist flexors

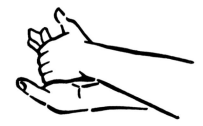

Starting position and instructions
Straighten your right arm, and with your left hand, take hold of the palm of your right hand below the knuckles and pull your right hand back into extension. Hold the stretch for 10 seconds and then repeat.

Variations
Placing the thumb of the left hand in the crease at the back of the right hand will localise the stretch to the area of the wrist.

Coaching points
There are seven small carpel bones within the wrist and this exercise will stretch all of the wrist, but will not isolate the stretch to a single bone. If a single joint is stiff, manual therapy from a physiotherapist will be required before the stretch is placed on.

Exercise 45 · Wrist abduction and adduction

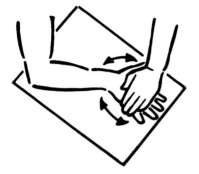

Starting position and instructions
Place the right forearm on a low table with your hand flat and fingers spread. Place your left hand over your right to prevent your hand from sliding on the tabletop. Glide your forearm from side to side encouraging abduction and adduction at the wrist.

Variations
Both abduction and adduction can be combined with a slight amount of flexion or extension to vary the stretch.

Coaching points
There is always more adduction (movement towards the little finger) than abduction (movement towards the thumb) available at the wrist.

Exercise 46 · Finger flexors

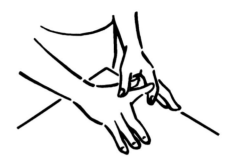

Starting position and instructions
Grip one finger of your right hand, placing your left thumb on the first metacarpophalangeal joint. Place the forefinger of your left hand underneath the right finger. Pull the finger back into extension. Repeat on all fingers.

Variations
Combining extension with abduction and adduction will vary the site of stretch.

Coaching points
Because of the leverage involved, the stretch must be slow and controlled.

Exercise 47 · Finger flexors and palm of the hand

Exercise 48 · Finger adductors

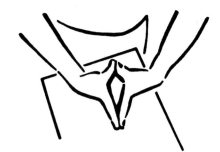

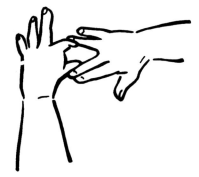

Starting position and instructions
Place the tips of yours fingers and thumbs together. Press your hands closer together to force your fingers and thumbs into extension. Hold the stretch for 10 seconds and then repeat.

Variations
Because the tissues being stretched are superficial, heat will increase the range of motion. The exercise can, therefore, be performed with the hands submerged in warm water.

Coaching points
Individuals who have extremely lax finger joints may find that their distal interphalangeal joint hyperextends. If this is the case they should start with the fingers flexed first and then stretch to the mid-position only.

Starting position and instructions
Place the right hand on a flat surface and place two fingers of the left hand between two of the right. Force the right fingers apart.

Variations
A small golf ball may be used between the fingers instead of the other hand. Pressing the golf ball closer to the web of the hand increases the range of motion obtained with the stretch.

Coaching points
Because of the leverage involved, the stretch must be slow and controlled. In individuals where the distal interphalangeal joints are hypermobile, a stretch may be placed closer to the finger web.

♦ Advanced ♦

Exercise 49 · Hip flexors and extensors (modified lunge)

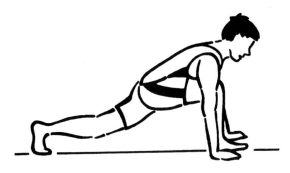

Starting position and instructions
Start with your feet shoulder width apart. Step forwards, leading with your right leg and lower your body towards the ground supporting your weight with your hands. Keep the right foot flat and the knee and foot in line.

Variations
Placing the hands inside the knee will increase the available range of motion.

Coaching points
Because full body-weight is being used, the exercise must be performed slowly.

Exercise 50 · Hip flexors (partner)

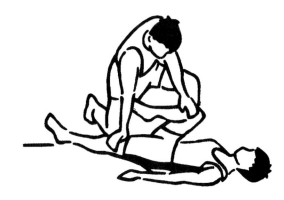

Starting position and instructions
Lie on the floor with your right hip and knee flexed. Your partner half kneels at your right hip. With their right hand they hold your left leg on the floor, and with their left hand they press your right leg into further hip flexion. This movement stretches the rectus femoris and iliopsoas of the lower leg, and the gluteals of the upper leg.

Variations
For those who experience pain in their knee, the partner's hand should be positioned on the under side of the knee.

Coaching points
Most individuals are asymmetrical so one leg may appear less flexible than the other.

Exercise 51 • Hip adductors – standing

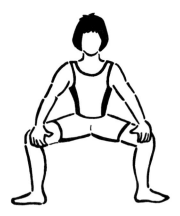

Starting position and instructions
Stand with your feet astride and toes pointing out. Squat down until your thighs are at 90°, placing your hands on your knees. Press with your hands to force your knees into further abduction.

Variations
Hold on to the ankle and press the knees apart with your elbows.

Coaching points
This movement is quite unstable so some individuals may find it easier to take their weight supported on a stool.

Exercise 52 • Hip adductors (partner)

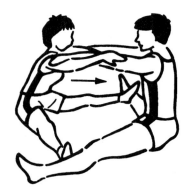

Starting position and instructions
Sit on the floor with your hips abducted. Your partner sits in front of you and places their stockinged feet on your inner shins. Link arms, and your partner presses your legs apart while pulling your trunk forwards. Hinge at the hips, keeping your spine aligned throughout the action.

Variations
Instead of pulling arm to arm, your partner places a towel around your waist and pulls your trunk forwards by pulling on the towel. This reduces the leverage on the spine.

Coaching points
There must be equal pressure between pressing with the feet and pulling on the trunk to increase flexibility. The aim of the trunk pull is simply to encourage pelvic tilt, moving the buttocks (ischial tuberosity) backwards in relation to the knee. When trunk flexion occurs the stretch has moved from the adductors to the trunk tissues.

Exercise 53 · Hip abductors (partner)

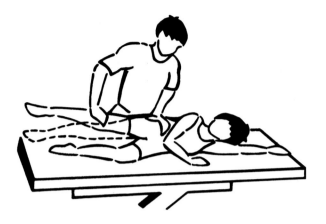

Exercise 54 · Hip rotation – lying (partner)

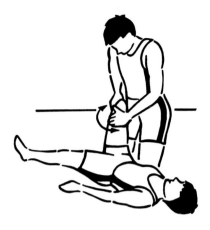

Starting position and instructions
Lie on a bench or the floor on your left-hand side; your partner kneels behind you at waist level. Your partner abducts and extends your right leg with their lower arm while fixing your pelvis with their upper arm. Keeping the pelvis stable (avoiding any side tilt) and pressing your right leg down into adduction, stretches the abductors.

Variations
Flexing the leg will emphasise the posterior portion of the gluteus medius.

Coaching points
Allowing even a small amount of pelvic movement will completely release the stretch in this exercise. You will only feel the stretch if you have tightness in the hip abductors of the upper leg.

Starting position and instructions
Lie on the floor with your partner kneeling on your right-hand side by your waist. Your partner flexes your right knee and hip, and presses it inwards and outwards encouraging rotation at the hip. This movement stretches the medial and lateral rotators of the hip.

Variations
Altering the angle of hip flexion will vary the stress on the hip rotators.

Coaching points
This exercise places stress on the pelvic joints so it must be used with caution following pregnancy.

Exercise 55 • Gluteals

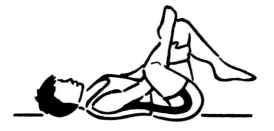

Starting position and instructions
Lie on the floor, flex the right hip and rotate it. Draw the left knee up, pressing the knee on to the right foot. Reach around the left knee and pull the knee towards the shoulder, forcing the right hip into external rotation.

Variations
Altering the angle of hip motion of the left leg will change the emphasis on the stretch.

Coaching points
This exercise also places stress on the pelvis so it is inappropriate after pregnancy.

Exercise 56 • Hamstrings and hip adductors – lying

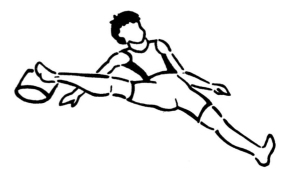

Starting position and instructions
Lie on the floor with both legs straight. Take your right leg into flexion and then out into abduction, aiming to rest it on the floor. Keep both shoulders and hips on the floor.

Variations
Place a small cushion or block under your leg to limit the full movement.

Coaching points
The subject must be strong to lower the leg under control, and under no circumstances should the leg be dropped rapidly towards the floor.

Exercise 57 · Hamstrings and hip adductors (splits position with stool support)

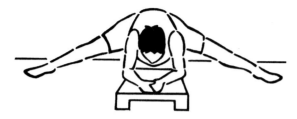

Starting position and instructions
Stand with your feet astride and then slide your feet apart to form a splits position. Flex your trunk at the hip and place your forearms on a stool to support your body-weight.

Variations
Place your feet on a shiny piece of paper (on a carpet surface) or cloth (on a wooden floor) to allow your feet to slide more easily.

Coaching points
The pelvis should remain above the hips throughout the movement and the body-weight must be taken on the forearms to reduce the stress on the knees. This exercise is unsuitable if you have had a knee liagment injury.

Exercise 58 · Hamstrings – sitting (partner)

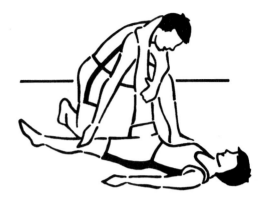

Starting position and instructions
Lie on the floor with straight legs. Your partner half kneels at your right hip and lifts your right leg, placing their hand over your knee to keep the leg straight. Your leg rests on your partner's shoulder and they lunge forwards, pressing your leg into further flexion at the hip.

Variations
Place a small pad on your partner's shoulder and a small rolled towel under your back to make the position more comfortable.

Coaching points
This exercise is most effective when used with PNF techniques.

Exercise 59 · Hamstrings – standing (partner)

Exercise 60 · Rectus femoris (partner)

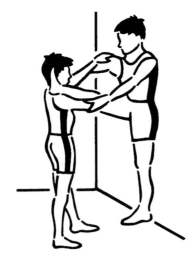

Starting position and instructions
Stand with your back to a wall; your partner stands facing you in a lunge stance, knees slightly bent. Place your right leg on your partner's right shoulder and take hold of their arms, keeping the leg straight. Your partner gradually straightens their legs, pressing your right leg into further flexion.

Variations
For extremely flexible subjects, your partner places their hands together and holds your foot as they press your hip into further flexion above their shoulder.

Coaching points
Stability is important, so if you find you are unstable during this exercise, hold on to the wall.

Starting position and instructions
Lie on the floor on your front and bend your right knee. Your partner half kneels at your right hip and places one hand in the small of your back, the other beneath your right knee. Your right foot rests on your partner's shoulder. By leaning forwards your partner presses your right leg into extension at the hip and flexion at the knee, while preventing any lumbar movement.

Variations
Increasing the amount of hip extension will emphasise the upper portion of the muscle.

Coaching points
Abduction of the hip should be avoided during this exercise.

Exercise 61 · Spinal rotation (using leg leverage)

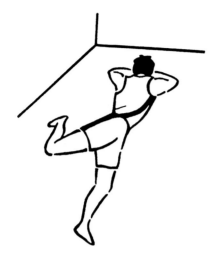

Starting position and instructions
Lie on your front with your arms supporting your head. Take your right leg up and across your body to touch the floor on the left, twisting your trunk and flexing the knee as the movement progresses. This exercise stretches the oblique abdominals.

Variations
Altering the degree of flexion at your knee and the extension of your hip will change the emphasis of the stretch.

Coaching points
Due to the weight of your leg, it should be lowered under control rather than forcing your spine into extension and rotation.

Exercise 62 · Lateral flexion and rotation

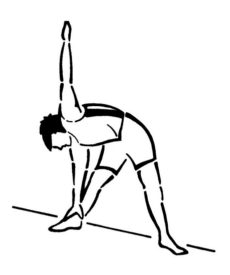

Starting position and instructions
Stand with your feet astride and turn your right foot out. Reach down towards your ankle with your right arm and point your left arm towards the ceiling to offer counter-balance. This exercise stretches the oblique abdominals and the quadratus lumborum.

Variations
Allow your upper arm to rest on your body to alter the stress.

Coaching points
The body-weight must be taken through your arm on to your ankle throughout the movement to reduce the leverage (stress) on your spine. If you have a history of lower back pain, you should only attempt this exercise under the supervision of a qualified instructor.

Exercise 63 • Anterior chest and shoulders

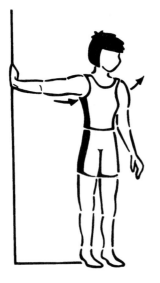

Starting position and instructions
Standing side-on to a wall, place your right hand on the wall at shoulder-height. Keeping your right arm straight, turn your feet to the left and rotate your body to the left, feeling the stretch across the front of your shoulder. This movement stretches the anterior deltoid, pectoral and biceps muscles.

Variations
Altering the height of the hand on the wall will vary the site of the stretch.

Coaching points
Because of the momentum involved in this exercise, the trunk twist must be slow and controlled at all times.

Exercise 64 • Anterior chest and shoulders (partner)

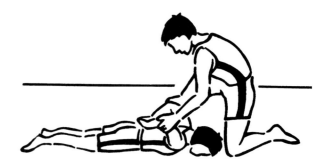

Starting position and instructions
Lie on the floor on your front with both hands in the small of your back. Your partner kneels at your head. Grasping your outer elbows, your partner leans back to pull your arms inwards and upwards. This movement stretches the anterior deltoid, pectoral and biceps muscles.

Variations
Pressing the elbows closer together, or leaving them further apart, will alter the exact site of stretch.

Coaching points
As with all partner stretches, the subject receiving the stretch must give feedback to lead the movement at all times.

Exercise 65 • Shoulder flexors

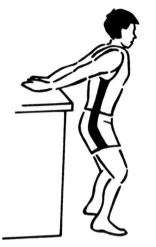

Starting position and instructions

Keeping yours arms straight, extend them behind you and place the back of your hands on a high table. Maintaining correct body alignment, bend your knees to lower your body, pressing your shoulders into further extension. This movement stretches the anterior deltoid, pectoral and biceps muscles.

Variations

Putting your hands closer together or further apart changes the muscle emphasis of the exercise.

Coaching points

In cases of shoulder dislocation this exercise should not be used: as the arm is forced back into extension the ball of the shoulder (head of the humerus) moves forwards in the joint, stressing the anterior structures.

Exercise 66 • Shoulder rotation (a)

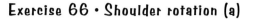
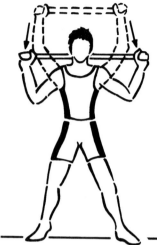

Starting position and instructions

Grip a bar above your head. Lower your arms so that the bar passes behind your neck, hold the position and then release. This movement stretches the medial rotators of the shoulder (subscapularis, deltoid, latissimus dorsi and pectoralis major).

Variations

A towel may be used instead of the bar provided the towel is held tight.

Coaching points

Assymetry in rotation is common, so one arm may be able to drop lower than the other.

Exercise 67 • Shoulder rotation (b)

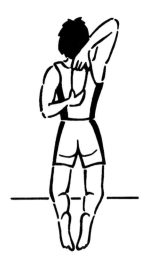

Exercise 68 • Forearm flexors

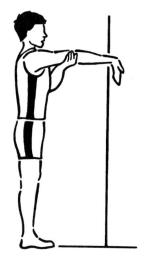

Starting position and instructions
Grasp a towel behind your back with your right arm placed behind your neck and your left arm in the small of your back. Move your arms up and down to lift and lower the towel vertically.

Variations
A broom handle may be used instead of the towel.

Coaching points
Assymetry in shoulder rotation is common, so the range of motion may differ when the arm placement changes.

Starting position and instructions
Place your right hand flat on the wall with your fingers pointing to the floor and your right arm straight. Hold your right elbow locked using your left hand. Lean your body-weight forwards, pressing the heel of your right hand into the wall.

Variations
Placing your hand higher up the wall will increase the stretch.

Coaching points
Releasing the elbow even very slightly will make the stretch less effective.

Exercise 69 · Thumb flexors and abductors

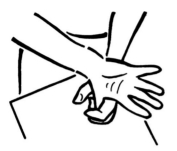

Starting position and instructions
Place your right hand palm up with your thumb extended. With your left hand, grip your right thumb from beneath and pull your thumb into extension and abduction.

Variations
Altering the exact position of the thumb will vary the site of the stretch.

Coaching points
Because of the leverage involved in this stretch, the force applied should be slow and continuous.

Chapter 9

Measuring Flexibility

Flexibility should be measured in order to:

• determine your existing range of motion;
• assess any muscle imbalance;
• chart your progress as you train.

Range of motion

When a muscle is more flexible than normal (hyperflexible), there is no need to stretch it; to do so could leave you open to injury. If a muscle is too flexibile, there may not be enough strength in the muscles supporting the joint to control the total range of motion: in such a case we say that hyperflexibility (greater than normal range of motion) has developed into instability (inability to control joint alignment through the whole available range).

Muscle imbalance

You will also need to assess the ratio of muscle flexibility on one side of the joint to that on the opposing side. When there is a marked difference in flexibility or strength between the two, muscle imbalance is present (*see* page 33) and it would be wrong to practise an overall stretching programme. This would simply allow the imbalance to continue, although your muscles, in general, would be more flexible. When imbalance is detected, the answer is to stretch only those muscles that are too tight, and to strengthen those that are too loose (flabby) and weak by exercising in the inner-range position. Once the imbalance has been corrected a general flexibility programme may be used.

Charting progress

Stretching is a long-term part of any training programme, so you will need 'goals' or targets to aim for. For this you will need to measure your flexibility and aim at improving it within a certain time. For example, you might aim at improving the range of motion of a joint by a certain number of degrees in a certain number of months; or aim to reach far enough to touch a certain point by a set date (for instance, Christmas or birthdays). Either way, the goals you set yourself must be specific and realistic. It is no good simply saying that you want to increase your flexibility, because this is too open ended: increase by how much, and in how long? Your goals must also be realistic: you may never be able to perform the splits if you are over 50 and very inflexible in the hip adductors. This really does not matter, provided that your degree of flexibility is appropriate to your age, body make-up and activity level. Remember, the right amount of stretching is the right amount for you as an individual. There is no competition – no winners and no losers.

♦ How to measure ♦ flexibility

Using a score chart

The score chart, illustrated in table 9.1 (*see* page 127), can be used as a test to measure your flexibility. Average values are quoted, but they are for general guidance only. If you have a specific problem which limits your flexibility you should see your physiotherapist.

You should perform a warm-up before testing any movement, and wear warm clothing to keep your body warm while performing the tests. Make sure that you perform the same degree of warm-up each time you measure your flexibility. The exercises are either active or static stretches (*see* page 46) and should be performed slowly and held in the stretched position. There should be no bobbing or bouncing actions which will give a deceptively high score. The instructions for each exercise are included in the table.

Clinical flexibility testing

The score chart can only give a rough, but still very useful, guide to flexibility. Where more precise measurement is needed, clinical testing is used. This accurately measures the angle of the joint at the point of maximal

stretch, and is called *goniometry*. A number of goniometers are available. The simplest is the *universal goniometer* (*see* fig. 9.1). This consists of a 180° or 360° protractor. It has a single axis and scale but two arms. One arm is held stationary, the axis of the goniometer is placed on the axis (centre) of the joint to be measured, and the two arms rest on the mid-lines of the bones either side of the joint. The joint angle obtained when stretching is read from the centre scale.

The *gravity goniometer* consists of a needle inside a fluid-filled container. The needle points downwards due to gravity and acts as a reference against which the joint range is measured. The goniometer is strapped on to the limb and a direct reading is achieved.

How to use the goniometer

Figure 9.1 shows the plan for a simple goniometer. Photocopy this, stick the copy on to a piece of firm card or plastic and cut out the shape. Fasten the two pieces together with a clip. The goniometer is now ready for use.

To take a reading, position point A over the centre of rotation of the joint. This is the point of the joint around which the movement appears to take place. Figure 9.2 shows the centres of rotation for the large joints. To maintain accuracy, the arms of the goniometer must be positioned parallel to the bones along the mid-line of the limb. Figures 9.3(a) and 9.3(b) show correct and incorrect alignment

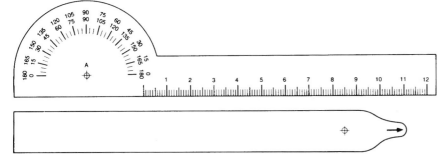

Figure 9.1 The goniometer

1 SHOULDER GIRDLE

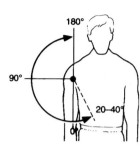

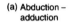

(a) Abduction –
    adduction

(b) Elevation –
    extension

2 ELBOW AND FOREARM JOINTS

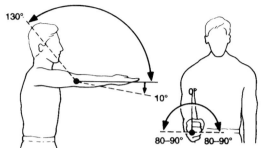

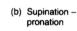

(a) Flexion –
    extension

(b) Supination –
    pronation

3 HIP JOINT

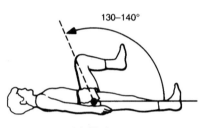

(a) Flexion

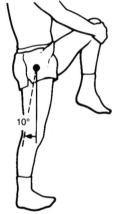

(b) Extension

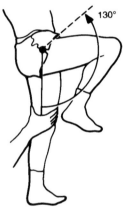

(c) Flexion

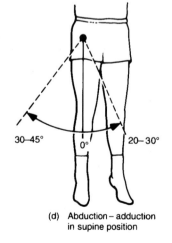

(d) Abduction – adduction
    in supine position

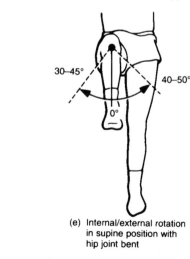

(e) Internal/external rotation
    in supine position with
    hip joint bent

Figure 9.2 Joint centres

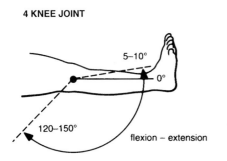

4 KNEE JOINT

5–10°

0°

120–150°

flexion – extension

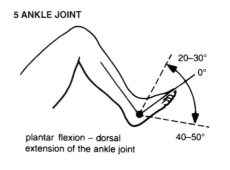

5 ANKLE JOINT

20–30°

0°

plantar flexion – dorsal
extension of the ankle joint

40–50°

Figure 9.2 cont. Joint centres

respectively. In figure 9.3(b) the upper arm of the goniometer is not aligned along the mid-line of the upper leg, so the reading obtained is lower, giving the appearance of a less flexible joint.

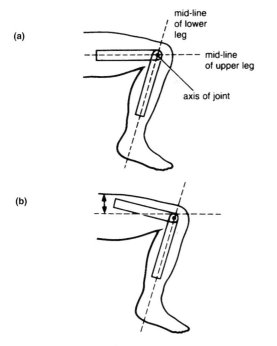

(a)

mid-line
of lower
leg

mid-line
of upper leg

axis of joint

(b)

Figure 9.3 Correct goniometer position: (a) correct alignment of goniometer with arms along mid-line of limb; (b) incorrect alignment gives appearance of reduced range of motion

♦ Accuracy in ♦ measurements

Spine and hip movement

When the spine is moving in combination with either the lower limb or upper limb, close examination is required to determine which joints are actually taking part in the stretching exercise. Tightness in the ligaments surrounding the hip means that once the hip has flexed beyond 90° the pelvis starts to tilt and the lower spine subsequently begins to flex. Total range of motion may be made up of movements at a number of joints. In figure 9.4(a) the individual appears to have long hamstrings because he is able to touch his toes. In fact, the hamstrings are short and the pelvis has stayed tilted back. The movement is occurring in the lumbar spine because the individual's spinal extensors are excessively flexible. In figure 9.4(b) the hamstrings are also short like those of the individual in 9.4(a), but the spinal extensors are of average length so the total range of motion is considerably reduced. In figure 9.4(c) the range of motion appears normal, but neither the hamstrings nor the spinal extensors is flexible. Instead the movement is coming from the thoracic spine which is rounding excessively.

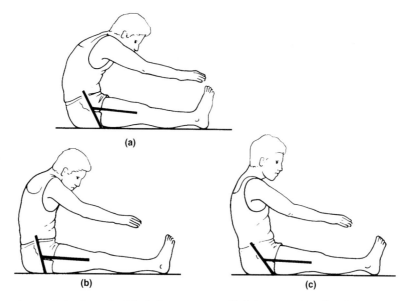

Figure 9.4 Sit-and-reach test – what is being measured? (a) excessive flexibility in spinal extensors; (b) excessive rounding of thoracic spine; (c) normal back flexion and short hamstrings

Pelvic and hip movement

Pelvic tilt is also an important factor in determining hip motion. In figures 9.5(a) and 9.5(b) the length of the rectus femoris is being measured. In figure 9.5(a) no pelvic tilt is occurring and the range of hip extension is seen to be limited. In figure 9.5(b) the same range of hip extension is occurring, but the anterior tilt of the pelvis, occurring at the same time, gives the appearance of an increase in total range of motion.

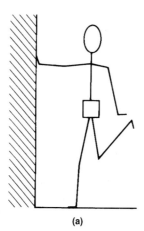
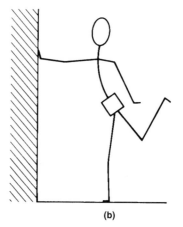

Figure 9.5 Pelvic tilt and hip extension

Table 9.1 Flexibility tests

Tick (✓) the box corresponding to your movement range following the guidelines listed below.
- Perform thorough warm-up before measuring your flexibility.
- Hold each stretched position for three seconds before measuring.
- Do not bounce into the movement.
- Average values will vary with body-size and body-type.

Test	Poor	Average	Good
1 Keep your straight leg on the floor and pull your bent knee towards your chest.	knee further than 15 cm from rib-cage	knee 10–15 cm from rib-cage	knee to rib-cage
2 Keep the soles of your feet together and press your knees downwards towards the floor.	more than 15 cm from floor	15 cm from floor	less than 15 cm from floor
3 Keep the knees locked and reach forwards towards the toes.	more than 15 cm from toes	10–15 cm from toes	touching toes
4 The lower leg is bent up to the chest and held still, the top leg lowers towards the ground.	above horizontal	horizontal	below horizontal
5 Stand 0.5 m from a wall. Lean forwards, keeping the feet flat on the floor and the knees locked	more than 60°	60°	less than 60°

Table 9.1 cont. Flexibility tests

Test	Poor	Average	Good
6 Keep the forehead and chest on the ground and lift the straight arm upwards.	less than 15 cm	15–20 cm	more than 20 cm
7 Reach behind the back and try to grip the fingers of the opposite hand.	fingers more than 15 cm apart	fingers 10–15 cm apart	fingers touching
8 Keep the arms straight and try to cross them over as far as possible.	cross at wrist	cross at elbow	cross at upper arm
9 Keep the foot flat on a stool and press the knee towards the wall.	more than 50°	40°–50°	less than 40°
10 Keep the knees together and bent to 90°. Allow the heels to drop outwards.	less than 70°	70°–90°	more than 90°

Table 9.1 cont. Flexibility tests

Test	Poor	Average	Good
11 Lock the arms flat out and measure the distance between the pelvic crest and the floor.	more than 10 cm	15–10 cm	less than 5 cm
12 Keep the arms flat on the floor and twist the trunk to allow the knees to lower towards the floor.	more than 10 cm	10 cm	0 cm
13 Keep the small of the back on the chair back and flex the spine (not the hips) maximally.	fingers to mid-shin	fingers to floor	flat hand to floor
14 Keep the feet flat and knees locked. Without leaning forwards or backwards reach down the side of the leg.	fingers above knee	fingers to knee	fingers below knee
15 Keep both legs straight and flex one hip as far as possible.	less than 90°	90°	more than 90°

Table 9.1 cont. Flexibility tests

Test	Poor	Average	Good
16 Abduct both legs while keeping the small of the back flat and the legs straight.	less than 90°	90°	more than 90°
17 Keep the knees together, and flex one knee maximally.	knee further than 10 cm from buttock	knee to 5–10 cm from buttock	knee to buttock
18 Keep the knees and ankles together throughout the test, and slowly sit back on to the heels. Measure the distance between the top (dorsum) of the foot and the ground.	greater than 5 cm	5 cm	flat

Spine and shoulder movement

Movement of the spine with the shoulder is also important. In figures 9.6(a) and 9.6(b) the range of shoulder elevation is being measured against the wall. In figure 9.6(a) the movement is seen to be limited, but in figure 9.6(b) there appears to be a greater range of motion. In fact, the range of motion at the shoulder is exactly the same in each case; it is the movement occurring in the spine which is greater in the second figure.

When measuring joint movement it is essential to limit the motion to a single joint. This can be achieved by looking closely at the body and repeating the movement to ensure accuracy.

♦ Using flexibility measures ♦ in research studies

When flexibility measures are being used as part of a research study, as discussed in Chapter 7, we need to be sure that the tests are both accurate and giving us the information that we think they are. Although a full discussion of experimental design and research techniques is not within the scope of this book, we will look at some fundamental processes. The interested reader is referred to Thomas and Nelson (1990) for further information.

Validity and *reliability* are two essential factors in measurement error. Validity asks the question, 'Does the test measure what it claims to do?', whereas reliability asks, 'Was each test of a batch the same?' Both are essential for maintaining the accuracy of stretching tests.

Validity

Take the example of a straight leg raise (SLR) action to measure hamstring length. We perform a certain number of stretches over six weeks and use the SLR to determine the best number of stretches for increasing hamstring flexibility. Is this a valid measure?

There are two types of validity: internal and external. *Internal validity* refers to the extent to which the results of a study can be attributed to the exercises (intervention) used. For example, if flexibility on the SLR does increase after six weeks, was this the result of our stretching programme or something else such as simply the passage of time? *External validity* is concerned with the generalisation of the results. In other words, are the changes that occurred in our experiment likely to

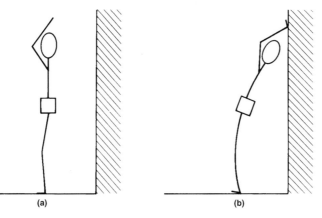

(a)   (b)

Figure 9.6 Spine and shoulder movements

occur outside the laboratory situation. Sometimes, an experiment may be so controlled that it no longer reflects what occurs in sport. For example, if we choose to measure the SLR lying flat and using a frame that fixed the pelvis and prevented the knee from bending to ensure accuracy, how does this compare to a football kicking action where the hamstrings are stretched in sport? Clearly there may be so many differences that the exercise is no longer the same as the functional action.

Internal validity

A number of factors may affect internal validity.

- **History** can affect internal validity if some other event occurred at the same time as testing which could have affected the results. For example, if we used students for our experimental subjects, some of them may have started a gymnastic programme at school at the same time as the experiment, and they may well have used hamstring stretching as part of their gymnastics, making it impossible to say whether our study, or the gymnastics, was responsible for any results obtained.

- **Maturation** refers to the passage of time. This is important when a study, especially with children, lasts for a prolonged period. For example, if we have a group of ten-year-olds and our study lasts for 2–3 years, are any results simply the effect of moving into adolescence and the flexibility changes that occur during this time?

- **Testing** will itself affect the results. Once we have measured hamstring length using the SLR, we have in fact stretched the hamstrings with the SLR test. The subjects have learned how to perform the test, and may be able to relax their muscles further.

- **Instrumentation** changes are also very important. For example, if we are using a goniometer (*see* page 123), the position of the goniometer and the type of goniometer used must remain the same, or the measurement obtained will be different, not through stretching, but through inaccurate measurement.

- **Statistical regression** is a tendency for factors to vary, especially if extreme measures (very flexible or very inflexible) are used. If we choose a group with very tight hamstrings for our study, we would expect them to vary in such a way as to move towards the average score. This is because all scores will vary with each measurement: sometimes a person is more flexible, and sometimes less. We are only measuring an average for that individual, and this average will constantly change.

- **Selection biases** encompass the number of factors involved in picking subjects for the study in the first place. For example, if we ask for volunteers for a flexibility study we may well get a lot of individuals who think they are flexible (we all like to show off!). Equally, those who stay with the study (six weeks is a long time) are likely to be those who are enjoying it, or have a particular reason to do it (perhaps it is a requirement for their college course).

External validity

When dealing with threats to external validity, remember that we are concerned with whether our results accurately reflect what happens in the real world.

- If we use a pre-test, i.e. we allow an individual to get used to the experimental setup before we test them, we may get **reactive effects of testing**. The subject would be prepared for the test and aware of what was coming. This would not occur on the sports field, for example, where the stretch would be performed during an exercise.

- We must also be careful that the way we select individuals for our study does not **interact** with the measurement we are using. For example, test results from subjects who know where their hamstrings are may differ from subjects who do not have this knowledge.

- If the results of our testing only occur in the laboratory but not in the real world, we are seeing **reactive effects of the experimental setup**. For example, we may choose to take a measurement with a very complex piece of apparatus that influences movement to such a degree that the movement is no longer similar to the one used in sport.

- If two or more stretches are given, the effects of one exercise may influence the other, and we have **multiple treatment interference**.

Reliability

Reliability is really the consistency of the results obtained from a series of tests. We can talk about reliability in terms of observed score, true score and error score. When we measure range of motion with a goniometer, for example, we are not measuring the real joint angle, because the goniometer is attached to the skin, and not to the bones. What we are seeing is an *observed* score. If we were to x-ray the moving joint and measure the bones directly, we would obtain the *true* score. The difference between these two, the real range of motion and the apparent range is the *error* score.

The error in a measurement may come from four main sources.

- **Subject** errors include things such as motivation, fatigue, and health. If, in our study, an individual injures their hamstrings, this will affect their flexibility and, therefore, the test results. Equally, a subject who is less motivated may not pull the limb as far as they would if they were practising an active stretch.

- **Test** errors may occur through lack of practice and familiarity with the results, for example, as well as through technique and lack of attention to detail. When a tester knows the value of a result, they may be able to influence it by over or under estimating a measurement. Equally, a poor standard of testing through lax positioning of a goniometer, for example, may produce considerable error.

- **Scoring** error is due to the selection of inappropriate measurement values. For example, measuring joint movement in single inches rather than degrees.

- **Instrumentation** error results when instruments are not calibrated, or they simply break down – something which happens all too often.

◆ Summary ◆

- We need to measure flexibility to know the current level of a client's movement range.
- Measuring flexibility enables us to judge if any muscle imbalance exists, and to chart a client's progress.
- Flexibility can be measured using score charts and measuring devices (goniometers).
- Angles obtained during measurement are compared to normal values and to the other side of the body.
- Measurements may appear accurate when, in fact, they are not. Exercises that combine movements of two body-parts simultaneously must be checked closely.
- Validity asks, 'Does a test measure what it claims to do?', while reliability asks, 'Was each test of a batch the same?'

Chapter 10

Stretching and Sports Injuries

♦ Tissue healing ♦

If you slip on a pavement and sprain your ankle, the body reacts immediately by starting a healing process. This process can be divided into three phases: *inflammation, proliferation* (sometimes called regeneration), and *remodelling*.

Inflammation

Following injury the inflammatory phase lasts between four and six days. The appearance of the body at this time reveals four classic signs: redness, swelling, heat and pain, which together lead to a loss of function in the injured body-part (*see* fig. 10.1).

- **Redness:** When tissues tear, small blood vessels are ruptured releasing blood into the surrounding area. Injured tissue-cells die and chemicals are released irritating the local tissues causing local blood flow to increase, which leads to the red appearance.

- **Swelling:** Changes in the concentration of fluids around the blood vessels cause watery fluid to leak out of them and into the surrounding tissues, giving rise to swelling. If the injury is close to the body surface, for example an injured ankle ligament, the swelling is readily apparent; if the injury is deeper in, however, the swelling may not be seen on the body surface, but only felt as pressure and stiffness.

- **Heat:** Increased metabolic activity from the inflammation causes heat, which is felt over the skin surface.

- **Pain:** The combination of pressure from the swelling, and chemical irritation from metabolic products causes pain.

With a minor injury the inflammatory phase may end in three days, but with more serious injuries inflammation can remain active for five or six days. When an injury occurs and the tissues tear, their tensile strength (capacity to stretch) immediately drops (*see* fig. 10.2). During the inflammatory phase, the strength of the injured tissues relies on clotted blood and tissue fluids so the injured area is very weak. Until the blood and swelling clears and new collagen tissue forms, the tensile strength of the area remains poor. During this time, we

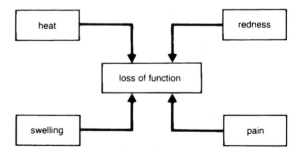

Figure 10.1 The signs of inflammation

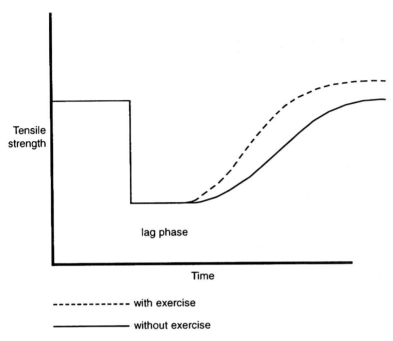

Tensile strength

lag phase

Time

- - - - - - - - - - - with exercise

———————— without exercise

Figure 10.2 Tissue strength following injury

will join the damaged tissues by forming a bridge.

The collagen fibres are laid down haphazardly, and if this orientation remains the scar formed will be very weak. To improve the strength of the scar, gentle movement should be performed, which will stretch the healing collagen fibres and cause them to line up in the direction of stress applied, making the eventual scar far stronger. The size of the collagen fibres also depends on regular movement: with exercise, larger and stronger fibres form and the fibres bond to each other, further increasing the tissue strength. Exercise, correctly prescribed, will therefore create a stronger and more suitable healing breach across injured tissues (this is represented by the dotted line on the graph shown in figure 10.2). Most of the collagen will have been laid down by 16 to 21 days after injury, so this is the time when stiffness will be greatest and stretching will be most effective.

say that the tissues are in their 'lag' phase where, although healing is progressing, tissue strength remains unalterred. Any stretching applied at this stage can easily disrupt the healing process and prolong the inflammation, making the total healing time longer.

Proliferation

Following inflammation, *proliferation* occurs. Within the injured area, the cells that were supplied by the damaged blood capillaries will have died and these must be removed if healing is to be effective. Removal of dead cells is the job of special blood cells that engulf the dead material and digest it. Once this has occurred, new capillaries start to grow into the damaged area, forming delicate granulation tissue. By the fifth day after injury a special form of tissue called *collagen* (*see* page 17) has started to form; this material

Remodelling

About 21 days after the injury, the *remodelling* phase begins. During this phase the amount of collagen produced is equal to the amount broken down. Although the total amount of collagen remains the same, the fibres overlap and form a mat of adhesions, which will stick to the surrounding tissues if movement is not performed. The collagen will also begin to shrink unless stretching exercises are continued.

♦ Time-scale for stretching ♦

As we discussed above, it is clear from the effect on healing that stretching is not appropriate immediately after injury for the following two reasons. First, the injured area is very weak and easily disrupted. Any amount of stretching could easily pull it and increase the tissue damage, which, in turn, will re-start the inflammation. Second, collagen tissue will not begin to form until the dead material produced by the injury is removed, so until that happens there is nothing there to stretch.

We can divide the post-injury period into two distinct phases (*see* fig. 10.3).

Acute phase

The first is the *acute* phase, from the day of injury to four days after. During this time the area is still inflamed, and our aim should be to minimise the effects of the injury. This may be achieved by using ice or cold water to slow down the metabolic rate, and reduce cell death from the low amount of oxygen present in the area. Swelling should be contained by using an elasticated bandage and the fitness of the rest of the body should be maintained by using exercises which do not stress the injured area.

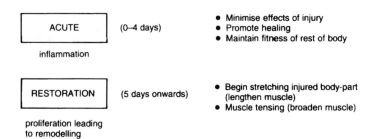

Figure 10.3 Acute and restoration phases of an injury

Restoration phase

After five days the inflammation will have subsided, and we enter the *restoration* phase. Stretching is needed to ensure that the collagen fibres of the injured tissue strengthen and face in the right direction to support the body-part. Strengthening exercises must also be performed to tense and broaden the muscles. This moves the muscle fibres apart and prevents them from sticking together.

♦ Classification of injury ♦

When muscles are injured we say they are *strained*; when ligaments are injured they are *sprained*. Both strains and sprains may be categorised into grades that represent the severity of the injury and the amount of tissue that has been damaged.

Ligament injuries (sprains)

Three grades of ligament injuries are used. Grade I sprains involve only slight tissue damage and the area is tender to touch, swelling is only slight, and the body-part moves almost normally. With grade II sprains, more ligament fibres are injured, local pain is more intense and movement is more limited. Grade I and II injuries are common when, for example, the ankle is twisted. Grade III injuries are far more serious because they involve complete rupture of the tendon. A skiing injury is a typical example of this type. There is considerable pain and swelling, and it is impossible to take the body-weight through the injured limb. These injuries often require surgery to repair the ruptured ligament, followed by intensive physiotherapy.

Muscle injuries (strains)

Muscle strains may be classified into four grades. Grade I (mild) strains involve tearing of only a few muscle fibres and subsequent local bruising. The area feels stiff for a few days and then clears up fairly quickly. Grade II (moderate) strains are more severe. A larger number of muscle fibres are injured, and injury occurs over a greater area. The muscle membrane (fascia) still remains intact, so bleeding is contained within the muscle and forms what is called an *intramuscular haematoma*. The area again feels tight, but this time a local raised area is felt over the bruising and when tensed or stretched the muscle gives pain. A pulled hamstring is an example of a grade I or II muscle strain. With grade III (severe) strains a larger area of muscle is affected. The muscle fascia is partially torn, and more than one muscle may be involved. Bleeding is more profuse, and it spreads over a larger area: because the muscle fascia has torn, blood spreads throughout the area causing skin discoloration. A typical example here is a 'dead leg', where bruising spreads from the injured thigh down into the knee and calf. The grade IV injury is a complete rupture. The muscle-ends contract and a distinct gap can be felt between the injured muscle fibres. In some cases a snapping sound may have been heard at the time of injury. Bleeding and swelling are considerable, and the muscle cannot be tensed up. This type of injury may require hospital treatment.

The classification of an injury is a guide to the period of rest and the amount of stretching that is required. As a general rule the stretching should not be painful, but you should feel that it is lengthening the muscle. Never force a stretch, and never exercise through increasing pain. If something is painful, and the pain goes away with stretching, that is fine. However, if the pain starts to increase, the stretch should be stopped.

♦ Stretching exercises for ♦ injuries

The following stretches are for general guidance only. If you suffer a sports injury, see a physiotherapist. The sooner an injury is seen, the better; if left without treatment, injuries can put you out of sport for far longer. In addition, minor aches and pains are often signs that something is going wrong with the body. If this is caught in time a more severe injury can often be prevented.

The sprained ankle

When you sprain your ankle, the most common injury is to a portion of the lateral ligament on the outside of the joint. This tissue limits plantarflexion, inversion and adduction of the foot. The easiest way to stretch this area is to cross the injured leg at the shin over the uninjured one, one hand steadies the lower leg on the injured side, while the other is cupped around the foot and ankle to pull it down, round and inwards. The stretch should be gentle and static.

Once this has been achieved, the next stage is to stretch the ankle actively by standing and rocking over on to the outer edge of the foot, or by walking on an inclined surface. This movement is controlled, but eventually faster actions must be used to develop agility in the ankle structures. This can be achieved by walking on an uneven surface such as soft ground or sand. You can also make your own uneven surface by placing four or five cushions on the ground and walking, and then slowly jogging, over them in bare feet. At each stage the action must be controlled so you don't feel that the movement is 'running away' with you.

Shin splints

Shin splints is a condition affecting the shin muscles, which are contained within compartments running alongside the tibia and fibula. With training, the muscles swell and thicken and as this happens the pressure within them increases. Because the muscles are contained within an inflexible compartment, they cannot bulge outwards, so they bulge inwards, cutting off their own blood supply. It is this reduction of blood flow and the build-up of acids within the muscles that causes pain. Stretching exercises can help some types of shin splints by preventing the muscles becoming short and tight.

On the front of the shin, the anterior compartment contains tibialis anterior and the toe extensors (*see* fig. 10.4). These muscles pull the foot and toes up into dorsiflexion. To stretch them, we have to press the foot slowly into plantarflexion immediately after running (*see* Chapter 8, exercise 21). Initially we begin kneeling with the feet flat on the ground. From this position we sit back onto the heels, pressing the feet into plantarflexion. To increase the stretch on the toes, place a folded towel on the floor beneath the toes to press them into flexion. Hold the position for 30–60 seconds to allow the muscles to 'give' gradually. Repeat the stretch five times after each run.

The pulled hamstring

When you tear a hamstring you may injure the muscle in its centre part (belly), or at the musculo-tendinous (MT) junction – the point at which the hamstring joins to the bones of

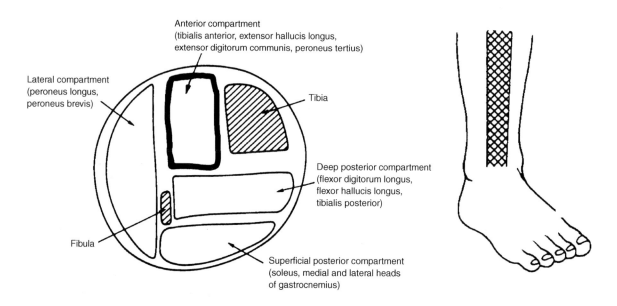

Figure 10.4 Compartments of the lower leg (Norris 1998)

the pelvis, or the knee, via the muscle tendon (*see* fig. 10.5). The difference between these two areas is that the MT junction does not contract, while the muscle belly does. As well as stretching, muscle-belly tears will need strength training to broaden the muscle and separate the muscle fibres to prevent them from sticking together. Injury to the MT junction often responds to stretching alone.

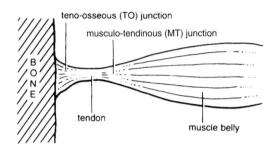

Figure 10.5 Areas of injury in a muscle

Because the hamstrings work over the hip and the knee, two types of stretches are necessary. First, the muscle must be stretched with the leg straight (*see* Chapter 8, exercise 4). Then, once adequate flexibility has been regained, the elastic strength of the muscle must be worked on. First stretch the muscle, then contract it rapidly from this lengthened position. To do this, lie face-down on a bench with the injured leg over the bench side so that the hip is flexed to 90°. A small (3 kg) weight is attached around the ankle. From the stretched position the hip is extended to pull the leg upwards against the resistance of the weight (*see* fig. 10.6(a)). The movement may be modified to use both the knee and the hip by training with a partner. The partner provides the resistance by pushing on the heel, and the movement starts with the knee and hip both flexed to 90°. From here, extend both the hip and knee simultaneously against resistance, hold the maximally contracted position for one to two seconds, and then lower the leg while maintaining tension in the

muscle (*see* fig. 10.6(b)). This controlled action progresses to spring jumping actions (*see* fig. 10.6(c)), moving from a flexed hip/knee position to a fully extended position.

To work the upper part of the hamstrings and the gluteals, we have to perform a posterior pelvic tilt against resistance. Functionally, the action involves lifting, so this can become a useful exercise. The action is called a 'hip hinge' or 'good morning' exercise (*see* fig. 10.7). Begin standing with your legs straight and a stick across the shoulders. Keeping the legs and back straight, bend forwards from the hips to 45°, and then return to standing. The action must move from the hip as a pivot

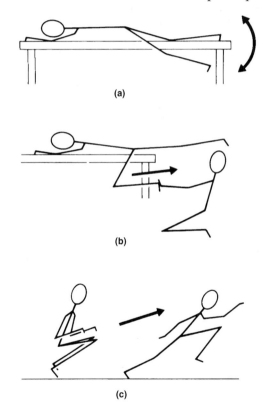

Figure 10.6 Combining strength and stretch of the hamstrings: (a) hip extension over side of bench; (b) combined knee and hip extension against partner's resistance; (c) sprint jumping

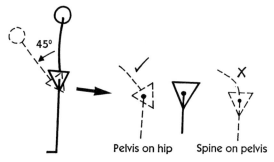

Figure 10.7 Hip hinge action

rather than from the lumbar spine: moving from the lumbar spine will dangerously over-stretch the lumbar tissues.

The swollen knee

When the knee suffers a minor injury it will swell and limit the movement of the joint. As the swelling clots and the injury heals, both the physiological movements and the accessory movements of the joint will be limited (*see* page 20). This means that the joint will lose its normal movement and its healthy springy feeling (joint play). Stretching into flexion and extension will help you to regain the physiological movements, but the accessory movements will only return if these actions are combined with stresses to the knee

that apply rotatory and shearing forces. These will work on all aspects of agility, and also help to build 'confidence' in the knee.

Start by standing with the feet shoulder width apart, step forwards and across with the uninjured leg so that the stress is taken on the injured knee. Step backwards and across to place the opposite stress on the joint (*see* fig. 10.8(a)). This action may be used as a side-step to perform a 'grapevine' action. Bending the knee further will increase the stress on the knee, and performing the action over a bench to bend the knee to near maximum will test the knee fully (*see* fig. 10.8(b)). Because these actions stress the knee considerably they must be carefully controlled.

When the rotation movement of the knee is limited, particularly after injury to the inner ligament (medial collateral ligament), this can be regained by twisting the tibia on the femur. A simple exercise is to place the foot up on a swivel chair so that the knee and hip are flexed to 90°. Turn the chair by twisting tibia and foot. As the foot moves outwards the tibia is externally rotated and the medial ligament is stretched. Gentle stretching of this type will make the ligament stronger by stressing and relaxing it to help the ligament fibres line up in the direction of the stress on the knee.

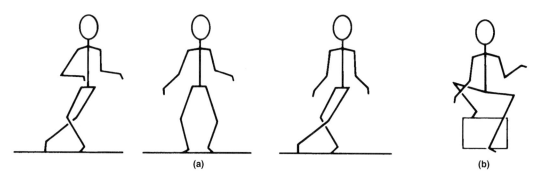

Figure 10.8 Developing agility in the knee: (a) 'grapevine' movement to place sideways stress on knee; (b) increasing range of movement

The 'kicking' muscle

Injury to the rectus femoris or the 'kicking muscle' is common in football. The injury usually occurs either when an ineffective warm-up has been performed, or towards the end of the game when fatigue sets in. Either way, stretching is needed to restore the length and spring of the muscle. Passive stretching is performed by simultaneously flexing the knee and extending the hip (*see* Chapter 8, exercise 5). Once the same range can be achieved on both the injured and the uninjured side, the elastic strength of the muscle must be worked on. The action is to move from a fully stretched position to a fully contracted position of hip flexion and knee extension. This is performed against a resistance which can be supplied by an elastic band, by a low pulley in a weight training room, or by a training partner (*see* fig. 10.9).

Groin strain

Groin strain is also a common injury in football, and in other sports which involve rapid sideways stretches while lunging or side-stepping. The adductor muscles of the hip attach to the lower part of the pelvis. The adductor longus, adductor magnus and adductor brevis all attach to the femur and have no action over the knee; gracilis, however, attaches to the upper part of the inner surface of the tibia, so it can also flex the knee during certain actions. This is important, because adductor stretches must be performed both with the knee flexed to take gracilis off stretch and tax the other adductors, and with the knee extended to stretch gracilis itself. Two exercises are useful.

In the first exercise (*see* fig. 10.10(a)) begin sitting on the floor with the soles of the feet together. Holding the feet with the hands, presss down on to the knees or thighs to force them into abduction.

The second stretch emphasises the gracilis. For this, lie on the back with the legs straight. Flex the right leg to 90° at the hips, keeping it straight. From this position the leg is abducted, aiming to rest it on the floor (*see* fig. 10.10(b)). Repeat using the left leg. In both exercises, PNF (contract–relax) stretching may be performed by lifting the legs against resistance (manual in the first stretch, gravity in the second) and them lowering the legs again to increase the range of motion. It is important for total rehabilitation of the adductor muscles following groin strain that strength training and stretching go hand in hand. As the rehabilitation period progresses, fast explosive actions (plyometrics) must be built in. This can be done usefully in a swimming pool with breaststroke type actions and using elastic tubing in the gym.

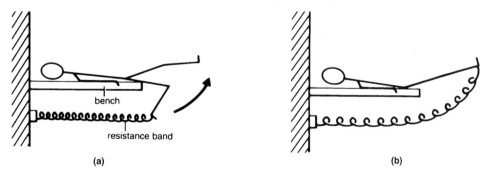

(a)   (b)

Figure 10.9 Stretch–contract of the rectus femoris: (a) fully stretched position (hip extension and knee flexion); (b) fully contracted position (hip flexion and knee extension)

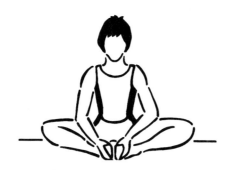

Figure 10.10(a) Hip adductor stretch for groin strain

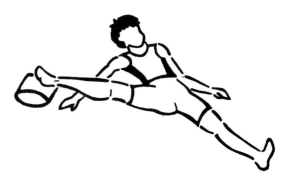

Figure 10.10(b) Hip adductor stretch for groin strain emphasising the gracilis

The dead leg

A 'dead leg' occurs when the quadriceps muscles of the thigh are severely bruised. This normally happens in rugby when a knee or head contacts the thigh at speed in a tackle. Blood vessels are ruptured and a large amount of blood is released into the muscle. The result is a large tense area within the muscle caused by a combination of blood and swelling. As the condition heals, the bruising tracks down through the muscle into the knee and calf. The athlete is unable to bend the knee because of tension in the quadriceps. The danger with this injury is that the release of blood can cause the area to calcify and form calcium bone salts within the muscle. If this happens it can be very serious, so stretching must be applied very cautiously under the supervision of a physiotherapist.

Initially, only active stretches should be used by lying prone and simply flexing the knee through the power of the hamstrings alone. Once 90° knee flexion has been obtained, very gentle passive stretches may begin by lying supine and pulling the heel up towards the buttock. A towel placed around the ankle makes the reach easier. When the range of movement increases further, and the pain and bruising subside, greater over-pressure can be used to stretch the quadriceps by kneeling and sitting back on the ankles. These quadriceps stretches are described in Chapter 8, exercises 20 and 21.

The calf and Achilles

When the Achilles is injured, calf stretches are performed with the knee flexed (*see* Chapter 8, exercise 7); when the calf is injured, it is usually the long gastrocnemius muscle which is affected and this is stretched with the knee straight. When this can be performed statically without pain, the following active stretch is used.

Stand on a 5 cm block (a thick book) and place the ball of the foot on the back edge. Allow the heel to lower down, keeping the knee locked: this will stretch the gastrocnemius. Starting from the standing position again, raise up on to the toes against your body-weight. Initially you should hold on to something to take some of your body-weight off the calf. Eventually, full body-weight may be used and the exercise can be speeded up until faster, more explosive actions are used to work the muscle for elastic strength.

The arch of the foot

In sports, such as the martial arts and some types of dance, which are carried out in bare feet or in very thin shoes, the amount of motion available to the big-toe joint can overstretch one of the structures which forms the arch of the foot. This structure, the *plantarfascia*, can become inflamed or damaged. If this happens, stretching should be employed once the injury has healed in order to restore flexibility. This can be achieved by plantarflexing the foot and flexing the toes simultaneously. The plantarfascia will stand out as a tight cord in the sole of the foot.

The ribs

The ribs may be bruised or cracked, for example in a rugby tackle, or when hit by the ball in hockey or cricket. When the injury has healed, stiffness often remains because the muscles between the ribs (intercostals) have tightened. To open the ribs and stretch the intercostals we need to combine overhead reaching actions with deep breathing. Twisting the trunk away from the painful area will increase the stretch still further. When performing this exercise be careful not to take too many deep breaths without a rest, because this could cause you to hyperventilate and become light-headed. Perform the exercise three times and then breathe normally for 30–60 seconds before trying again.

The frozen shoulder

When the shoulder is injured, it will swell and the joint capsule will fill with fluid. This will cause the capsule to tighten, eventually limiting the movement of the whole joint. Due to the shape of the capsule certain movements will be limited more than others. In the case of the shoulder, lateral rotation (placing the hand behind the neck) becomes more limited and painful than medial rotation (putting the hand behind the back). The rotation movements may be regained by trying to touch the fingers together behind the back (*see* Chapter 8, exercise 67). Joint play may also be regained by holding on to an object and leaning back to pull the shoulder along its length and apply traction (*see* fig. 10.11(a)). Alternatively, sit sideways on a dining chair and hang your arm over the chair back. Place a thick towel over the chair back to pad the armpit area. Grasp some thing in the hand to provide a traction force, and pull down on the stiff arm with the other arm to give overpressure (*see* fig. 10.11(b)).

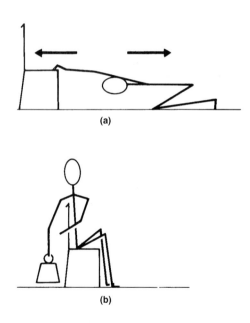

Figure 10.11 Self-traction in the shoulder joint: (a) hold object and sit back on your heels; (b) hang arm over chair back

Tennis elbow

In tennis elbow the muscle most commonly affected is the one which extends the wrist (extensor carpi radialis longus). This muscle will become tight and must be stretched by flexing the wrist while keeping the elbow locked out. If the elbow is allowed to bend even slightly the stretch will be taken off. A simple exercise is to stand facing a wall, and to straighten the elbow and keep it locked with pressure from the other hand. Place the back of the hand of the injured side against the wall and lean forwards to press the wrist into flexion (*see* Chapter 8, exercise 43). Performed correctly, this stretch can be felt up the whole arm and into the elbow.

Because the extensor carpi radialis longus also abducts the wrist, a further stretch may be placed on the muscle by adducting the wrist at the same time as flexing it. This is achieved by standing with the arm by the side, pronating the forearm and flexing the wrist (*see* fig. 10.12). Take hold of the hand and press the wrist into further flexion and adduction, pulling the wrist towards the little finger (ulnar deviation).

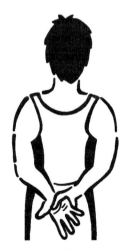

Figure 10.12 Stretching the extensor carpi radialis longus muscle in tennis elbow

Tennis elbow often involves the nervous tissues travelling through the elbow. The upper limb tension test movements described on pages 77–8 are usually very relevant. Re-strengthening the forearm extensor muscles is also vital.

Wrist injury

Following a wrist injury, such as a severe sprain or fracture, most of the movements at the wrist will be limited. To regain these, three exercises are important. The first two are performed with the hand flat on a table top. Initially the hand is placed palm down on the table surface, with the wrist crease at the table edge. The uninjured hand is placed on top of the injured one, and the elbow is moved up and down to produce flexion and extension of the wrist (*see* fig. 10.13(a)). The leverage provided by the forearm combined with the weight of the body provides overpressure at end-range for the static stretch.

For the second exercise the hand is moved into the centre of the table, so that the whole forearm is supported, and again the uninjured hand holds the injured one flat against the table surface. The elbow on the injured side is moved from side to side, sliding over the table surface to perform abduction and adduction of the injured wrist (*see* fig. 10.13(b)). Finally, the arm is held at 90° flexion with the elbow close into the side of the body, the injured forearm supported by the cupped uninjured hand. A stick is held in the hand, and pronation and supination performed. Aim to move the stick into a horizontal position (*see* fig. 10.13(c)).

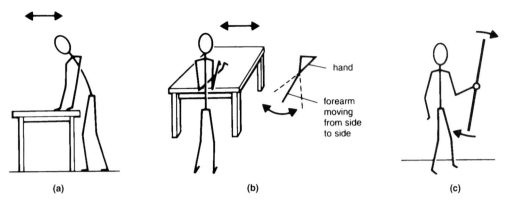

Figure 10.13 Wrist mobility exercises

Finger injuries

Finger injuries are common in many sports and caused either through trauma, for example in martial arts and football, or from overuse, for example in rock climbing. Where swelling is profuse, movement can often become limited very quickly, so stretching is vital. As the structures of the hand and fingers are very delicate, the stretching should be applied 'little and often' as a general rule. Three or four shorter bouts per day being better than a single long bout.

The movements are flexion, extension, and abduction. All performed with manual overpressure. For flexion, the finger is bent to its maximal extent, and then gripped on the proximal and distal phalanx. Pressure is exerted to try to bring the finger tip to the underside of the knuckle. With extension, the movement must be isolated to each individual joint. One finger is placed proximal to the joint to fix it while the other is placed distal to the joint to force the movement. For both of these movements, the exercise is best performed after soaking the hand and fingers in comfortably hot water for 15–20 minutes. Abduction is performed with the hand supported on a flat surface. The fingers are abducted and overpressure placed using two fingers of the opposite hand. The pressure is maintained for 20–30 seconds and then released.

◆ Summary ◆

- Inflammation shows as redness, swelling, heat and pain.
- Proliferation is the stage of tissue regeneration.
- During proliferation dead tissue is removed by white blood cells and new tissue forms. Controlled movement is needed to encourage correct tissue placement.
- When injured, ligaments sprain and muscles strain.
- Stretching forms a vital part of injury recovery.

Chapter 11

Sport-specific Stretching

♦ Designing your own ♦
programme

In the majority of sports there is a central core of muscles which require stretching. Most sports involve some type of running action: this may be repeated running (marathon); single step running or lunging (badminton); or small bursts of speed (football). In each case the muscles used are similar, but the intensity of use, and the range of motion will differ. While the running action forms the basis of motion, the throwing action frequently involves either a ball (throw and catch) or an implement used to strike an object (racquet or bat).

Superimposed on these two basic sports movements are actions specific to the individual sports themselves. For example, the double-arm throwing action used in football differs considerably from the action of throwing the javelin, while the striking action of bat on ball in cricket is different from that of hitting a ball with a tennis racquet.

Therefore, to build up a comprehensive stretching programme for sports, we need to choose exercises which cover both the core sports actions and the specific sports actions. By analysing which muscles are used in an action, we can estimate the patterns of muscle tightness that are likely to occur for each sport. Developing a stretching programme in this way can achieve two things. First, sports actions will be more efficient because we maintain a high range of motion. As we have seen on page 24, if a muscle is contracted from a comfortably stretched position the amount of force achieved is greater than if a muscle is contracted from a shortened position. By stretching, we are therefore enhancing sports performance. Second, by preventing excessive shortening in general, and muscle imbalance in particular, we are maintaining optimal joint alignment. This provides a foundation for good biomechanics and balanced joint loading, increasing the likelihood of injury prevention.

♦ Movement analysis of ♦
core sports actions

Running

Running differs from walking in that when we walk we have at least one foot on the ground at all times; when we run we literally jump from foot to foot, so there is a stage when both feet are off the ground and the body is airborne. For this reason, running may be divided into two component phases, *stance* and *swing* (*see* fig. 11.1).

In the stance phase the foot is on the ground, and the body is decelerating. The muscles are working eccentrically to slow the body down and absorb shock through the whole of the lower limb. At the moment when the foot strikes the ground, the body-weight is

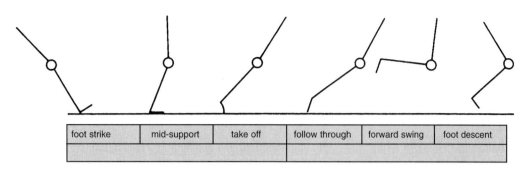

foot strike	mid-support	take off	follow through	forward swing	foot descent

Figure 11.1 The running cycle (Norris 1998)

taken through the heel. As the body-weight moves forwards the foot flattens to absorb the shock, and finally the foot pushes with the toes to accelerate the body once more and propel it forwards. The forward action signals the start of the swing phase when the foot is off the ground. The limb is now accelerating and being catapulted through the air.

During heel strike, the anterior tibial muscles work to stop the foot slapping down on the ground, while the posterior tibials stop the foot from flattening too much. Tightness in either of these two muscle groups can be a cause of shin pain in runners. In mid-stance the knee is bent slightly and the quadriceps work to provide the spring in the legs, while the hip abductors support the pelvis and prevent it dipping down at the side. Tightness in these muscles at this stage of running is one cause of pain at the side of the leg and knee (or 'runner's knee'). As the heel rises and we begin to push off from the floor, the hamstrings rapidly extend the hip while the calf muscles plantarflex the foot. Both provide the thrust in running. If either muscle is tight it is more likely to tear during sudden lunging or sprinting actions. During the swing phase, the hip flexors lift the leg through. These may become tight and therefore more susceptible to injury, but usually

any excessive tightness or shortness will affect the lumbar spine.

Stretches for running
Sports involving the running action will require calf, Achilles and anterior tibial stretches. In addition the hip flexors, hamstrings and quadriceps should be stretched together with the abductors. Sprinting actions will require more attention to the hamstrings, while kicking actions will need stretching for the rectus femoris. Endurance running will need stretching for the ilio-tibial band (ITB) and anterior tibial muscles, in particular, to protect against overuse friction injuries to these areas.

Throwing

In many sports the throwing mechanism is very similar. A javelin throw and an overhead shot in tennis may seem very different, but both have three phases (*see* fig. 11.2).

Initially there is the *cocking* phase, in which the arm is held up and back in preparation for the strike. The shoulder is abducted and externally rotated, the elbow flexed, and the wrist extended. This position stretches the anterior shoulder structures and shoulder rotators and can place considerable stress on

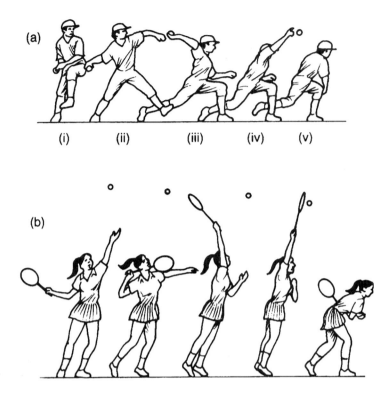

Figure 11.2 (a) The throwing action: (i) wind-up – athlete positions himself for the throw; (ii) cocking – lead leg moves forwards, arm moves backwards stretching body; (iii) acceleration – body drives forwards leaving arm behind; (iv) deceleration – object released, elbow continues to extend and shoulder to internally rotate; (v) follow through – trunk and lead leg show eccentric activity to dissipate energy; (b) similarity of throwing action to tennis serve (Norris 1998)

the medial ligament of the elbow. As the arm is pulled forwards into the striking position, it enters the *acceleration* phase. The body and shoulder lead the movement, coming forwards and leaving the arm behind, which pre-stretches the shoulder tissues. The shoulder flexors then contract rapidly with the shoulder rotators and elbow extensors to simultaneously bring the arm forwards and in. The acceleration phase takes place as a whipping action and so places considerable stress on the elbow structures. As the hand is flung forwards the arm enters its final phase, the *follow through*. The object being thrown is released from the hand, and the elbow extends rapidly. This places considerable stress on the bony knuckle of the ulna (olecranon process) as the elbow locks out.

Stretches for throwing
Sports involving any type of throwing action will require stretches to the anterior shoulder structures, the shoulder rotators and the elbow flexors. In addition, because of the single-arm nature of throwing, stretching must ensure symmetry between the two upper limbs.

♦ Movement analysis of ♦ specific sports actions

To know which additional stretching exercises are required, we need to analyse a particular movement used in a sport to find out which muscles it is affecting.

It is usually the muscles stretched by large movement ranges that we are concerned with, because these will be the ones needing stretching exercise: when throwing the javelin, for example, the shoulder and elbow of the throwing arm travel through extreme ranges so they will need stretching. The amount particular muscles are used must also be noted: those used powerfully are likely to shorten and require additional stretching. For example, the pectorals and anterior deltoids are used powerfully when performing bench-press actions in weight training so they tend to become very short.

Postures used in a sport are also a clue to the stretches which may be needed. Prolonged activity in a particular posture will cause the body to adapt by lengthening muscles on over-stretched joints, and shortening those other joints not moved through an adequate range. In cycling, for example, the stooped position of the thoracic spine can give rise to stiffness and pain in this area.

The movement analysis process may be divided into four stages (*see* table 11.1).

- **Stage one:** Initially we look at the movement and decide in which plane the movement mainly occurs (*see* fig. 1.11, page 10). This will give us an idea of the types of movement used. Abduction and adduction occur in the frontal plane, while flexion and extension occur in a sagittal plane, and rotation in a transverse plane.

- **Stage two:** Once we have an idea of the type of movement involved in an action, we must decide which joints are moving and which remain still. For example, in a trunk movement, is the hip moving as well? Does the pelvis move on the spine or on the hip, or both?

- **Stage three:** After the joints we consider the muscles which would ordinarily work to bring about the actions we have seen, for example the muscles which flex the hip. We then need to determine if these muscles actually *are* working during the sporting action we are looking at, and to do this we must palpate (touch) the muscle.

- **Stage four:** Finally, the fact that a muscle is working during a movement does not necessarily mean that it warrants stretching. To determine this, we need to know the range of motion (*see* page 10). It is only when a muscle is taken through a greater range than normal (full outer and full inner range, rather than simply mid-range) that we need to stretch it.

Table 11.1 Analysing movement in sports actions

Plane of movement	Frontal – abduction and adduction Sagittal – flexion and extension Transverse – rotation
Joints moved	Major motion only
Muscle action	What normally brings about action and what is acting now (palpation)?
Range of motion	Does range warrant stretching?

We will look at three examples from common sports to illustrate the movement analysis method: a football kick, a forehand shot in tennis, and a golf swing when teeing off. The recommended stretching exercises are from Chapter 8.

The football kick

When a kicking action is performed the movement analysis is as follows.

- The movement occurs in both a *sagittal* plane and a *frontal* plane because the kick moves forwards and across the body.

- This movement will be *flexion* and *adduction of the hip, extension of the knee,* and *plantarflexion of the ankle.*

- Some transverse plane motion may also be seen as the trunk *rotates* on the standing leg.

- The muscles involved in this action would, therefore, be the hip flexors and adductors, knee extensors, and ankle plantarflexors. In addition, the abductor muscles of the standing leg will stabilise the pelvis to stop it from dipping, and the trunk muscles will control the trunk rotation brought about by the momentum of the swinging leg.

- The range of motion of both the hip flexors and adductors is greater than normal, as is the range of the plantarflexors. The twisting of the spine would only be greater than normal in a less active individual who is beginning or returning to play.

The stretching exercises to choose, therefore, would be for the hip flexors, hip adductors (including gracilis) and calf muscles. Exercises 6, 12 and 14 would be appropriate.

The forehand in tennis

In an average tennis forehand shot the movement analysis is as follows.

- The left leg steps across the right to bring the body to face right (*right trunk rotation*).

- The right hand is raised (*abducted and extended*) to shoulder level with the elbow and wrist partially extending.

- The foot action is one of *dorsiflexion*, stretching the calf.

- The combination of trunk rotation and shoulder abduction/extension is usually rapid, though not of extreme range.

- Stretching exercises for the chest and shoulder should, therefore, be combined with power training for this area. The calf/achilles and wrist extensors are taxed considerably in all racquet sports through repetitive actions, so they too will require stretching.

Exercise 63 is appropriate for the chest/shoulder while exercises 7 and 43 are useful for the calf/achilles and wrist extensors.

The golf swing

In a typical golf swing (teeing off) the movement analysis is as follows.

- The body is angled forwards on the hips (*pelvis anteriorly tilted on the hip*) and the knees and hips are slightly flexed.

- The trunk is twisted (*rotation*) to the right on the semi-flexed leg.

- The arms are brought across the body to the right, raising the elbows to shoulder level and taking the hands over the right shoulder. To do this, the right shoulder *externally rotates*, and the left *internally rotates*, and these movements are reversed during the follow through.

- The trunk movement and the momentum of the combined body and club are taken through the semi-flexed knee, and considerably rotation occurs, slowly during the wind-up, and much more rapidly during the swing and follow through.

- The areas of concern are the combined movements at the trunk (flexion and rotation), which occur at speed and through considerable range, and the rotation at the knee. Both sets of movement are considerably greater than the normal movement ranges encountered in everyday life.

Trunk rotation stretches, pelvic tilt rehearsal and hip rotation movements are all important, with exercises 25 and 54 being appropriate. In addition, postural re-education may be required if an individual angles the body forwards through trunk flexion alone, with little movement of the pelvis on the hip.

◆ Summary ◆

- Running and throwing are core skills in many sporting activities.
- There are four stages to movement analysis: establishing the plane of movement, finding which joints have moved, determining which muscles are working, and finding the range of motion.

References

Adams, M. A., Hutton, W. C. and Stott, J. R. R. 1980, 'The resistance to flexion of the lumbar intervertebral joint', *Spine*, 5: 245–253

Astrand, P. O. and Rodahl, K. 1986, *Textbook of Work Physiology*, McGraw-Hill, Maidenhead

Bandy, W. D. and Irion, J. M. 1994, 'The effect of time on static stretch of the flexibility of the hamstring muscles', *Physical Therapy*, 74(9): 845–52

Barnard, H., Gardner, G. W., Diaco, N. V., MacAlpin, R. N. and Kattus, A. A., 1973, 'Cardiovascular responses to sudden strenuous exercise. Heart rate, blood pressure, and ECG', *Journal of Applied Physiology*, 34: 883–92

Bergh, U. 1980, 'Human power at subnormal body temperatures', *Acta Physiologica Scandinavia*, 478 (supplement): 1–39

Bergh, U. and Ekblom, B., 1979, 'Physical performance and peak aerobic power at different body temperatures', *Journal of Applied Physiology*, 46: 885–9

Butler, D. S., 1991, *Mobilisation of the Nervous System*, Churchill Livingstone, Edinburgh

Ekstrand, J., Gillquist, J., and Lilzedahl, S. S., 1983, 'Prevention of soccer injuries. Supervision by doctor and physiotherapist', *American Journal of Sports Medicine*, 11: 116–20

Enoka, R. M., 1994, *Neuromechanical basis of kinesiology*, Human Kinetics, Champaign, Illinois, USA

Etnyre, B. R. and Abraham, L. D., 1986, 'Gains in range of ankle dorsiflexion using three popular stretching techniques', *American Journal of Physical Medicine*, 65: 189–96

Gleim, G. W., Stachenfeld, N. S. and Nicholas, J. A., 1990, 'The influence of flexibility on the ecconomy of walking and jogging', *Journal of Orthopaedic Research*, 8: 814–23

Godges, J. J., MacRae, H. and Longdon, C., 1989, 'The effects of two stretching procedures on hip range of motion and gait economy', *Journal of Orthopedic and Sports Physical Therapy* 10(9): 350–7

Halbertsma, J. A., van Bolhuis, A. L. and Gloehen, L. N., 1996, *Archives of Physical Medicine and Rehabilitation*, 77: 688–692

Johns, R. J. and Wright, V., 1992, 'Relative importance of various tissues in joint stiffness', *Journal of Applied Physiology*, 17: 824–8

LaBan, M. M., 1962, 'Collagen tissue: implications of its response to stress in vitro', *Archives of Physical Medicine and Rehabilitation*, 43: 461–6

Li, Y., McClure, P. W. and Pratt, N., 1996, 'The effect of hamstring muscle stretching on standing posture and on lumbar and hip motions during forward bending', *Physical Therapy*, 76: 836–45

Magnusson, S. P., Simonsen, E. B. and Kjaer, M., 1996, 'Biomechanical responses to repeated stretches in human hamstring muscle in vitro', *American Journal of Sports Medicine*, 24(5): 622–8

McNair, P. J. and Stanley, S. N., 1996, 'Effect of passive stretching and jogging on the series elastic muscle stiffness and range of motion of the ankle joint', *British Journal of Sports Medicine*, 30: 313–8

Millar, A. P., 1976, 'An early stretching routine of calf muscle strains', *Medicine and Science in Sports and Exercise*, 22(3): 632–41

Moore, M. A. and Kukulka, C. G., 1991, 'Depression of Hoffman reflexes following voluntary contraction and implications for proprioceptive neuromuscular facilitation therapy', *Physical Therapy*, 71: 321–33

Nicol, C., Komi, P. V. and Horita, T., 1996, 'Reduced stretch–reflex sensitivity after exhausting stretch–shortening cycle exercise', *European Journal of Applied Physiology*, 72: 401–9

Norris, C. M., 1998, *Sports Injuries. Diagnosis and Management*, Butterworth Heinemann, London

Rosenbaum, D. and Henning, E. M., 1995, 'The influence of stretching and warm-up exercises on Achilles tendon reflex activity', *Journal of Sports Science*, 15: 481–4

Safran, M. R., Garrett, W. E., Seaber, A. V., Glisson, R. R. and Ribbecsk, B. M., 1988, 'The role of warm-up in muscular injury prevention', *American Journal of Sports Medicine*, 16(2)

Sullivan, M. K., Dejulia, J. J. and Worrell, T. W., 1992, 'Effect of pelvic position and stretching method on hamstring muscle flexibility', *Medicine and Science in Sports and Exercise*, 24: 1383–9

Taylor, D. C., Dalton, J., Seaber, A. V, and Garrett, W. E., 1990, 'The viscoelastic properties of muscle-tendon units', *American Journal of Sports Medicine*, 18: 300–9

Thomas, J. R. and Nelson, J. K., 1990, second edition, *Research Methods in Physical Activity*, Human Kinetics, Champaign, Illinois, USA.

Warren, C. G., Lehmann, J. F. and Koblanski, J. N., 1971, 'Elongation of rat tail tendon: effect of load and temperature', *Archives of Physical Medicine and Rehabilitation*, 51: 465–74

Webright, W. G., Randolph, B. J. and Perrin, D. H., 1997, 'Comparison of nonballistic active knee extension in neural slump position and static techniques on hamstring flexibility', *Journal of Orthopedic and Sports Physical Therapy*, 26: 7–13

Recommended Reading

Abdominal Training by Christopher M. Norris A & C Black, London 1997)

Anatomy and Human Movement by N. Palastanga, D. Field and R. Soames (Butterworth Heinemann, Oxford 1944)

Anatomy, Palpation and Surface Markings by D. Field (Butterworth Heinemann, Oxford 1994)

Back Stability by Christopher M. Norris (Human Kinetics, Champaign, Illinois 1999)

Human Movement Explained by K. Jones and K. Barker (Butterworth Heinemann, Oxford 1996)

Joint Structure and Function by C. C. Norkin and P. K. Levangie (F. A. Davies, Philadelphia 1992)

Muscles. Testing and Function by F. P. Kendall, E. K. McCreary and P. G. Provance (Williams and Wilkins, Baltimore 1993)

Neuromechanical Basis of Kinesiology by R. M. Enoka (Human Kinetics, Champaign, Illinois 1994)

Sports Injuries, Diagnosis and Management by Christopher M. Norris, second edition (Butterworth Heinemann, Oxford 1998)

The Complete Guide to Strength Training by Anita Bean (A & C Black, London 1997)

Weight Training, Principles and Practice by Christopher M. Norris (A & C Black, London 1993)

Useful Addresses

British Association of Sport and Exercise Sciences
114 Cardigan Road
Headingley
Leeds LS6 3BJ
tel 0113 289 1020

British Association of Sports Medicine
BMA House
Tavistock Square
London WC1 9JR
tel 0171 387 4499

Chartered Society of Physiotherapy
14 Bedford Row
London WC1R 4ED
tel 0171 242 1941

English Sports Council (North West)
Astley House
Quay Street
Manchester M3 4AE
tel 0161 834 0338

Fitness Professionals
113 London Road
London E13 0DA
tel 0990 133 434

National Coaching Foundation
same address and telephone number as
British Association of Sport and Exercise Sciences

National Sports Medicine Institute
c/o Medical College
St Bartholomew's Hospital
Charterhouse Square
London EC1M 6BQ
tel 0171 251 0583

Norris Associates
1 Barkers Lane
Sale
Cheshire M33 6RP
tel 0161 972 0512
website: http://www.norris.ndirect.co.uk

The Exercise Association
Unit 4, Angel Gate
City Road
London EC1V 2PT
tel 0171 278 0811

UK Sports Council
4th floor, Walkden House
3–10 Melton Street
London NW1 2EB
tel 0171 380 8003

Index